FRANCESCA LIA BLOCK

Guarding the Moon

A Mother's First Year

Moon

francesca Lia Block

HarperResource

An Imprint of HarperCollins *Publishers*

Library of Congress Cataloging-in-Publication Data

Block, Francesca Lia.

Guarding the moon / Francesca Lia Block.— 1st ed.

   p. cm.

Summary: Author Francesca Lia Block meditates on the challenges and gratifications of being a new mother.

ISBN 0-06-621367-3

1. Block, Francesca Lia. 2. Authors, American—20th century—Biography. 3. Pregnant women—United States—Biography. 4. Mothers—United States—Biography. 5. Mother and infant—United States. 6. Motherhood—United States. 7. Childbirth—United States. I. Title.

PS3552.L617 Z467 2002   2002068757

813'.54—dc21

[B]

Typography by Alicia Mikles

1 2 3 4 5 6 7 8 9 10

For Jasmine

New

· THE BIRTH OF THE MOON ·

*I*n a hospital room overlooking a twinkling, winking sleep of city I am stumbling. I am gripping onto the backs of chairs and onto my husband's shoulders that ripple as if trying to absorb my pain. I am crying out as my mother whispers softly to me, as if I were her baby again, her baby for the last time. The thunder through my pelvis is the truest sensation of life I can remember experiencing. Finally my body feels as if it is achieving what it had been insisting on since the first eggs came. I understand why I have been so hungry, why I have raged, why I have hurt myself trying to find love, why I have felt as if I would shatter if I did not find it. Now I prepare to shatter as I believe I was meant to all along. R. Carlos Nakai plays his flute on the stereo. The music is melancholy, windy, spanning deserts and skies burning red, spanning a universe of stars. The music is the shudders of pain that are telling me why I was born.

This goes on through the night. When the sky begins to pale and the city no longer looks like an enchantment of lights, the doctor comes to tell me I am still only three centimeters dilated and this could go on another ten hours or so, leaving me too exhausted to push. I decide to give up the startling, stunning education of the pain and get an epidural. The pain is preparation, an initiation into the selflessness and challenges of being a mother. And yet, Creation created these ways to alleviate the pain, too—created balms, potions, relief. I lie on my side as the soft-spoken anesthesiologist administers the drug. I am swept into a lullaby sleep tasting of lemons and sugar, smelling of lavender and almond oil, sounding of flutes, and feeling like the silk that is spun on the moon.

I wake fully dilated and begin to push. The impatient doctor, unabashedly eager to get to his weekend plans with his son, yells at me to bear down. I do so, hard enough that blood vessels burst in my face. My mother and husband are on either side of me, speaking gently, feigning calm. I am slow and numb below the waist. It seems to go on forever. Finally I reach down between my legs and feel where my body is splitting open to let my daughter's head emerge. It is slippery and hard and round. It is my daughter's head. The moon herself. That is when I fully awaken and see God. I cannot tell you any more than this. I announce to everyone, even my hurried, distracted doctor, that I see God. The universe cracks open and light pours into me, out of me. I push and scream to Creation. She emerges. In one split second I witness the transformation that is life. This never happened before. My father died behind a closed door.

But now my baby comes. Everything has changed.

She is laid upon my breast, slick with blood, her body tiny and still curled in the shape of my womb, her tucked-up froggy feet, her head perfectly round and smooth. She is whimpering and I speak softly into her Buddha ear. I tell her how much we love her. I tell her how we have waited for her forever. How grateful we are that she has chosen us. How we will do everything to make her happy. How she is our great treasure. My tears spill over us.

I weep in a different way when they take her away from me to wash her. I wonder how I will bear being without her even for moments. It is as if the best part of my body has been severed and swept off to be cleaned, swaddled, and topped with a pink knit cap.

When she is gone I feel clumsy and weak,

incompetent. I don't even know how to diaper a baby yet, let alone nurse her. I am choked with worry and grief that she is not with me. But then they bring her back.

Miss Pink gazes up at me with the heavy-lidded smoke-and-sea blue eyes that seem to stretch across her entire face. Her body molds to mine, as if we still share nerves, blood, excretions, sensation, emotion. I remember the umbilical cord, much thicker and bloodier than I would have imagined. I only got to glimpse it for a second before it was cut, leaving us separate. Now only our sweat makes us stick together.

But I feel fearless. With love. We are one again for now.

Crescent

· MOON MILK ·

*T*he fear begins again.

In the womb it was so easy to nourish Baby. Now I wonder about pain, if there will be enough milk; are my nipples too small? The lactation expert rushes in, eager to get on with her Easter vacation, and asks impatiently if I have taken breast-feeding classes. When I say no she gives me an irritated smirk and proceeds to manipulate Bubela into the awkward "football hold." I tense, imagining my darling whisked away to be given formula while my breasts dry up.

Instead, a few hours later, with the guidance of a real lactation expert, my mother, Baby Girl is feasting peacefully. Milk seeps through my clothes; jets squirt into her mouth. I can almost see how it makes her grow as she drinks, makes her turn pink pearl. She looks up drunkenly, nose rose, eyes dazed stars, bubbly mouth. She drinks until my breasts hang empty and I have to eat ravenously to fill them—vegetable soup, watermelon slices, and rice milk/almond/banana shakes. Then she wants more, squawking with delight, panting like a pup, curling and uncurling her toes, anchoring my elbow between her ankles, rolling her eyes with pleasure, smacking her cherry-pie lips. Later on, Milk Maiden begins to smile while she nurses, her mouth curving up tenderly around my nipple and her eyes sparked with mischief as she strokes, pinches, and scratches my waist and plucks at the fabric of my shirt, snapping it back against my body.

There is pain, too; my raw nipples feel like fragile silk, ready to tear off, or like hot coals, sizzling at the tips of my breasts. I apply gobs of lanolin until all my clothes are stained, but nothing helps. Maybe the painful tug near my heart is a way to relieve the buildup of so much love; it has to spill this way. Pain is grounding; it brings me back to reality where I have to be to raise a girl. It keeps me in safe shoes, although I long for my pale blue platform sandals. The glasses that I used to avoid wearing are now placed securely on the bridge of my nose so I don't miss a loose button that might choke a baby, a pin that might poke. Without pain, especially during those first days after her birth, I'd be floating out there on sunset clouds, ice cream, and daisies. Pain keeps me on mother earth. It makes me *become* mother earth with her ravaged survivor's body.

The pain lessens as my nipples toughen, thicken, but over time I begin to feel the nursing breaking down my body in other ways. I was told that in the yoga tradition breast-feeding is considered the equivalent of running five miles each time you do it. I am always hungry, my bones feel miniature and brittle, I have practically no libido—everything thinned where during my pregnancy there was voluptuousness. I am getting deeper grooves chiseled around my eyes from lack of sleep. I sit squinting at my computer as I try to finish a book for my editor, my vision getting worse every day. My hair, which was thicker than ever while my baby grew inside me, is falling out steadily. Strands of it end up gripped firmly in Bambina's fists as if she is planning on making a nest or a wig. I imagine myself as a bald, sexless stick figure, crudely stitched together, groping blindly in the dark.

Meanwhile Bebe is getting even more beautiful and luminous. It is as if I am sacrificing the fullness of my body for her gorgeous plumpness, my hair for the peach fuzz halo sprouting on her head and the dark eyelashes that dust her cheeks, my desire for the way she grasps my waist and chuckles with such sweetness that I feel a jolt of love in the pit of my stomach. Everyone who meets her gasps, reaches out for her, sighs. Men in shops and restaurants ask if she is married yet. One particularly unpleasant leering one says he wishes she were twenty-five years older. Friends I never used to see come over every week just to hold her. They say they feel healed by her presence, transformed by her smile. My brother, who has always been a bit reserved with his affections, in spite of my constant desire to win him over, brings her seven bears in hand-knit caps and sweaters and puts her picture by his bed. My husband calls her "Gawgeous," tells her he is madly in love with her, and sings, "She's the most beautiful girl in the world," over and over.

I think of my first miscarriage, how I collapsed to the floor sobbing, my springer spaniel trying to find a way to comfort me—finally too frightened by my screams to come near. I was screaming for my child. Maybe her spirit heard and decided to come, to find me, to be born. For this I can sacrifice my hair, my vision, my desire, everything. I see my death but I am not afraid now; for the first time, perhaps, I feel alive.

When I had the second miscarriage six months after the first, my mother told me, your baby will come, she will hear how much you need her and come to you. I thought, this isn't right, shouldn't she be the one who needs me? I should be the one with everything to give. But the truth is I needed her wildly.

Once I got mastitis and my breasts were balls of swirling flame swinging from my chest. I woke in the night crying and called the doctor. I was told that what would relieve and heal this was to nurse, nurse, nurse your child. This seemed wrong—that somehow she might get sick with the infection, too. I lifted Sugar Plum Fairy from the bed and felt the chill of her tiny hands pressed against my burning flesh like healing blossoms. At first it hurt more when she sucked, and I sobbed; but after a while the ducts opened and the milk spilled out again, my breasts cooled. It was like the night I went out into the garden, to pray to the moon to heal me. I breathed the heady night-blooming scent that could have been moonlight, and opened my body to the opalescence. Even as I suckled the nourishing milk from the moon I felt her beams gathering my pain and pulling it out of my body. Not taking it in to make her ill, but knowing just what to do with it.

This is my daughter. Giving as she receives.

· HOLDING THE MOON ·

I feel as if I have been called on to guard the moon herself. A moon with dimples and a tiny crooked grin. A moon with the sweetest scent emanating from the soft spot on the top of her round head—a smell sweeter than honey or flowers. How do you do this? How do you safely carry the moon around on this earth?

When we first brought Teenie Wee home from the hospital, it seemed shocking that we were allowed to take her outside, put her into the backseat of the car, and drive through such loud, bright, crowded streets. I sat back there with her, trying not to think of car crashes and how she was so little that her car seat straps barely stayed on her shoulders. I wished, then, that I was a marsupial with a pouch, hopping happily, hippily through a jungle. After giving birth my body was so different that it wouldn't have seemed odd to have a new flap of skin formed on my abdomen, a soft sling that appeared overnight for cradling the little one. But there was nothing except my still distended, now empty uterus. And months later I still want a pouch.

The car seat is just not natural in any way. This struck me most when we left the wee-ist one sitting in it asleep one night on the bed. Illuminated by light from the television and the blue globe lamp, crunched down with her features pressed together beneath a little man-in-the-moon cap, the creature in the seat looked like an elf or young alien who had been captured in a net in a forest among the roots of a gnarled tree and imprisoned in this contraption with its straps and buckles.

Even the starry night sky print doesn't help the car seat seem less sinister. There is a huge WARNING sign right near Babela's head about how DEATH may occur if the seat is not used properly; this makes me crampy-sick to my stomach every time I see it. The car seat has a strap that must be snapped into a slot between two pearly chubette thighs. It takes a lot of pressure to do this and makes a loud, painful sound. Every time I snap Bunny in I cringe and wince, imagining what might happen if I pinched her legs with the metal. When I lug the heavy seat out to the car I hear my birdish wrist bones clicking, threatening to collapse. Finally the car seat is in and then I must drive. I find that I hold my breath at almost every intersection, in spite of my yoga training. I feel nauseous at each left turn, waiting to make sure I can see everything in front of me before I creep forward, causing people behind me to honk their horns. I say an incantation to keep me calm. Because Fuzzy Wuzzy must face the back of the car, I can glimpse only the downy top of her head and hear the soft jingling of one of her stuffed guys—purple rhino, yellow giraffe, or striped and multicolored whoozit—as we go along. When she falls asleep her head lolls forward like a flower on a slender stem and I now have a new worry. Will her neck hurt? I know that kangaroos do not have to fret about such things.

The carriage looks sturdy and safe, but it, too, is covered with warning signs, and as we go down curbs I always pray that the straps have not somehow come loose and that the wheels are still secure. There is something strange, any-way, about setting out with your young riding far in front of you, the first to brave traffic, rather than contained against your body. Our spaniel, Vincent Van Go Go Boots, accompanies us proudly along the narrow sidewalks, keeping perfect pace. We dodge poisonous oleanders, dog shit, garbage, mud. We nervously try to catch the eye of each driver at stop signs. Once I startle so much at a car coming toward us that the driver decides to be funny, inching up slowly toward the carriage while I stand like a headlight-stricken deer. He laughs, "What, you thought I was going to hit you?" Even the sun seems to be playing mean games, peeking in on the moon baby skin at every opportunity. Instead of the calm my walks used to bring to me and Vin, we return home exhausted and tight. I remember when I was pregnant and we would walk up steep hills, go on two-hour treks down streets without sidewalks, climb the many flights of stairs among the gardens of palm, bougainvillea, and riotous six-foot-tall wildflowers. Now we can only take one route and it is not a meditation but an obstacle course. Our baby usually falls asleep, though. I peer down at her through the little sunroof in the top of the carriage and see two glimmering bluebells slowly close, rose feet stop kicking, bud fists no longer reach out to grab the cherries on the shade blanket. So this is my flower garden now. The best one even though I can't stroll through it but only peek at it like the magic worlds inside a sugar Easter egg.

My mother says that when I was a baby there were none of these contraptions; I used to ride in a little pink plastic seat in the car, or on her lap; there were no straps or belts or heavy high-tech carriers. But even the most natural, age-old baby-carrying devices seem daunting to my weakened body.

I have a cream-colored cotton Guatemalan Maya
wrap, but I can't get the hang of it. The tattooed
yoga goddess who sold it to me did an impres-
sive demonstration, tossing it over her shoulder,
making it look so easy, but when I use it, my
bundle wiggles and wriggles and writhes and I
end up just carrying her in my arms. This is wonderful; my arms feel her warm weight and my
skin absorbs her sweet smell. My food digests
easily and my body temperature regulates. And
yet I worry when I am trying to use one arm to
open a jar of vitamins or water a plant, is my
hold on her secure enough? In the first week,
when I was wretched with no sleep, staggering
to the changing table, my hands gripping the
treasure, I saw horrifying flashes of accidents.
The room spun with fatigue and worry. The
world was all sharp corners and edges, germs
and poisons, carcinogens. Doorknobs and cabi-
net edges seemed to come to life in the swirling

night, little demons of destruction that I must battle.

Why was I so haunted? I felt raw with guilt that I even envisioned my beloved in danger. I have often lived in fear, punishing myself with harsh judgments, obsessions, and near-starvation as, perhaps, a way to ward off the loss of my loved ones. This fear, now, cannot be distanced. But such a heightened, vivid, hallucinatory fear had its own weird purpose. In my exhaustion, which might otherwise have made me less diligent, the cringing fear kept me brilliantly, shockingly alert. I don't run from wild animals, but I still feel jolts of adrenaline that just fester and strain my heart. Now here is fear with a purpose, and I try to honor and respect it even as I tell myself that a good mother is always calm. Maybe I can learn to love fear, too. It will make my arms strong even when they shake with fatigue. In a strange way, wrapped around love—love's guardian—it will be my pouch.

Cannibal mamas in Mommy and Me yoga threaten to devour the miraculous toes of their babes. My baby giggles giddily when I put my mouth around her feet, pretending to savor her piggies. My mother says she thinks it is an instinct to take the little ones back inside where they are safe. The womb is even better than the pouch, but I know I will have to let Tinkletoes go out in her car seat, her stroller, eventually on those pink silk pouch feet, into the world with all its dangers.

My husband and I joke that no one can touch her but us until she is twenty-five and ready to marry my friend's blue-eyed son, who, when I was enormously pregnant and feeling completely unattractive, put his hands on my belly and crowed huskily, as if seeing straight through that wall of flesh, "The baby is cute!" We tell her that we will have lots and lots of fun until then, watching videos, eating take-out Japanese, and playing behind a locked gate in the garden—we'll even build her a fountain and gazebo covered with roses. But we know our fantasy won't last long. Already little boys reach out to touch her hand, so pudgy that it looks as if someone tied a little string bracelet around her wrist.

Once she was inside of me, tucked up, upside down, kicks and hiccups, my own secret. Once she was a flicker of heartbeat on the ultrasound screen and then a little shadow-baby there, with a spine like a fish's, like a fern's, scratching her elbow, sucking her thumb, and revolving to look out at me with the two sparks of light in her face.

Now she belongs to this place, to the night that rises out of the throats of the purple flowers, to the pale dawn singing the white flower of her name.

I never want to let go. We all strive to protect her. Our bodies make a fortress around her. When I set her in her crib at night I imagine that I am leaving my heart there to watch over her like a guard dog—fierce, jumping at every sound.

Vincent Van Go Go Boots has never been a guard dog. I found him at a gas station in the desert when my car broke down. He had been there a week, and the attendant was planning on taking him to the pound that day. When he ran up to me and looked into my eyes, I knew that he was mine. We were each other's. On the drive home he kept his heavy brown-and-white pony head in my lap, let me play with his topknot tuft of hair, and listened as I whispered names to him, to see which one made him respond. None did, but I saw an exit sign: VINCENT; he has four white boots—voilà.

He has been with me through heartbreaks and joyful delirium. He watched possessively as my husband and I first kissed each other. He has seen me crawl on the floor screaming with pain, weeping into his furry neck. We have walked miles and miles together, reveling in air and leaves and sunlight. We have both been very ill and nursed each other back to health.

Vincent has taught me a great deal about how to nurture another creature, given me confidence to have a baby, I think, since he is the only young thing I have ever had in my care. And he has cared for me, too, placing his head on my chest to comfort me when I am sad, rushing to my side when anyone raises his voice to me.

But as protective as he is, he has hardly ever barked or growled. Until now.

After the Love Dove was born he began sleeping facing the door, barking ferociously at the mail-man, lunging at the screen, baring his teeth. It makes me proud and also afraid. How much he has changed. We all have.

Vincent had always been the baby of the family. Now, none of us can be babies. We have all given up cuddling and complaints; there just isn't time. Vincent has stomach problems; my husband gets headaches and backaches; I experience pains in my neck and my gut, infections, a general sense that my body is falling apart. But we can't be too concerned. All of us are guardians now.

I worried about Vincent at first. When we brought Pinky Pie from the hospital he looked at me with such sadness, especially when he wasn't even allowed to kiss her. The first night he stole a piece of chocolate; it can be deadly for dogs. He threw up for days afterward and moaned in his sleep.

But now Vincent has someone new to love and be loved by, a companion to help protect Baby.

One day we saw a dog running with that frantic look of the lost. When I called her she came right into my arms. The tag around her neck was blank, and no one responded to the FOUND signs I put up or the ad in the newspaper. A number of animal rescue people I called suggested that I take her to the pound so her owner would have the chance to find her. I gave her vitamin C and echinacea to ward off kennel cough and forced myself to follow this advice.

But her first night at the pound, I suddenly had to lie down, curled on the bed, sobbing uncontrollably as if I could feel her in a cold cell, in cages smelling of death, coughing hoarsely for hours, her tail thumping the cement until the tip bled.

When I finally was able to claim her she recognized me immediately and began barking, leaping a few feet in the air like a circus dog. She came home and lay on Vincent's bed, making herself into as tiny a ball as possible.

The next day she began barking incessantly until the neighbor came over to complain, barked so that my child levitated a few inches in the air with the startle. The dog jumped up on me when I held my baby, making me fear scratch marks on tiny chubby thighs. She stole Little's brown-and-white stuffed dogs and a pink rabbit with ears twice as long as its body.

With my husband gone for twelve or sometimes fourteen hours a day at work, my baby almost always in my arms, and Vincent vomiting in the house every few weeks, I thought I wasn't able to welcome another family member. But no one else seemed to want this middle-aged, cat-chasing beagle mix, and I couldn't turn her away.

Maybe some of our bond had to do with the fact that we are both mommies. The vet said she'd probably had a couple of litters of pups. Her distended, swollen nipples, especially prominent against a starving rib cage, reminded me of how my own felt. Maybe this identification is what made me keep her after our attempts to find a home for her failed.

I wanted to call her Willow because of her sad eyes and long legs, but my husband chose Thumper because of her manic tail. Maybe I agreed because part of me didn't want to get too attached; Thumper certainly wasn't a name I'd choose for my baby and I couldn't have this fur girl as my second daughter.

Sometimes I think she was sent to us as much for Vincent as for any other reason. He finally has his soul mate. He no longer looks at me with the haggard, haunted expression when I leave the house. Two Dogs, as I call them, lie in the exact same positions on their velour animal-print beds and follow each other around all day. Every so often Vincent will lick his friend's ears lasciviously and paw her until she retreats into a corner, bewildered but never angry. Once she lay on her back for him, her paws tucked almost demurely to her chest, while he licked her unabashedly displayed nipples, belly, and rear and then stood over her, territorial and shuddering with excitement. Once she even tried to lure him, sniffing his groin and pawing his hind legs. Sometimes she licks the cyst on his eye with the intensity of a healer in a trance. He succumbs to her like a newborn animal being groomed by its mother. I have noticed that his eye looks much better now.

After my daughter insists on hearing the facts of life as demonstrated by Two Dogs, I will tell her the whole Mama Dog story. I'd like to keep some of it from her, just as I'd like to keep Hiroshima and the Holocaust and slavery. But I will tell her.

When I went to pick up Thumper from the pound, I was afraid to look at what was in the cages around me. But I made myself look. I thought, it is the least I can do for them—look, feel, cry, maybe tell their story. A small dog quarantined alone in a cage in the shelter vet's tiny office, his muzzle one red mosaic scab, his eyes still full of a mad hope. Heaps of golden puppies escaping into sleep and one another's warmth. Kittens with oozing eyes and skeletal bodies, they looked more like birds than felines. Noble old beasts hardly able to fit in their cages. Animals shaking, wailing, and pleading. Then I'll tell my moonbeam how we brought our mama doggy home.

I'll tell her that when she cried, Thumper came running. Any sound outside made her spring to attention; she blocked doorways with her body. While I breast-fed she looked at me with tender longing and a certain understanding in her sad, lopsided beagle-ish mug. When my mother came over, Thumper ran to her and pressed her snout against her breast, as if trying to nurse. My baby reached out to softly pat Thumper's sleek black head, stared at her with delight. I'll tell her how, at first, Thumper stole the brown-and-white stuffed dogs as if remembering her babies. But then she seemed to realize that though her babes were gone, she was now part of a team to raise this one. She joined us in our mission to protect the pink-toed princess who lives at our center— the heart of all of us, the little love goddess who makes my nurturing endless, my love tireless, my arms so full of her sweetness but somehow, because of her, always able to welcome more.

Mama Doggy still shakes and cries in her sleep sometimes; perhaps she cries for her pups. Maybe they are running zigzag through the streets or caged in a shelter or worse. I hold my pup curled against me, wanting to keep her there forever.

· LULLABY MOON ·

Sleep is another separation. How can I sleep? Every time I look at my daughter, my heart throbs with wakeful excitement and the need to guard this precious, delicate being. A being whose fourth toe on both her feet was so fragile at birth, almost threadlike, the piggy that had no roast beef. A girl with skin so thin I see rivulets of veins flowing beneath her scalp and on her eyelids. There is even one prominent vein beside her left eye, as blue as the eye; people often ask if she has bumped herself there. But no; she is translucent.

The first night in the hospital I had to put her down in the clear plastic case beside my own narrow bed and the cramped cot where my mother slept like our fragile guardian angel. After trying to close my eyes for a few moments, I opened them again to see that my baby had turned her knit-capped head to look at me. Her eyes flew like bluebirds; they reminded me of the goddess eyes I'd seen during healings I'd experienced in my life, a pair of light tilted eyes accompanied by the chime of finger cymbals and a shiver in my spine. I told myself, she is ours, she is here. I took her in my arms again and didn't sleep the rest of the night. At five in the morning I called my husband—who had gone home to be with Vincent—to make sure it was real. I had sat propped up for hours, terrified I'd crush or drop this dream dreaming in my arms.

When we got home from the hospital I was afraid to let her sleep between us. What if she was suffocated by our pillows or comforter? What if she slid down between bed and wall? Could we roll over her? My husband woke from nightmares, patting the bed, thinking she was stuck between the quilt and duvet cover. And yet, she wouldn't sleep in her white wicker basinette at our bedside; she always cried there. I scooped her up and nursed her, then sat propped against the pillows while she slept in my arms and I dozed dizzily, trying not to go into a deep sleep myself in case she fell. After a visit to the pediatrician I was reassured and placed her between us where she lay, soles of her feet together like a yogi, arms flung over her head in a gesture of hallelujah abandon, the "Exalted One" as my husband calls her. But ever since then I have only had a couple of unbroken nights.

Everything everyone said was true about the zombielike march of fatigue. Still, I didn't think sleep deprivation would make me feel psychotic. All the devils I wrestled with, and often conquered, in my dreams before were now unleashed to finish their battle on my unsuspecting psyche all day long. I was haunted by phantom shards of pain—humiliation, rejection, betrayal, disfigurement, dismemberment, disease, death. The one night that my daughter slept all the way through I dreamed of escaping from Hitler with her.

I thought I might find comfort in the crook of my husband's arm where I used to nestle when I felt sad or afraid, my head against his runner's heart. But we never lay this way anymore. Instead our baby slept between us. For a while she would turn to her papa, press against him and once, sick with lack of sleep, I remember feeling a shock of loneliness that I no longer had him, nor the secret mystery girl curled in my uterus.

And yet, maybe, the greatest comfort is a baby who needs comforting, who accepts my comfort. Each evening we nurse and she falls asleep against my heart. Almost every night at exactly eight thirty she thrusts out her lower lip, wrinkles up her face; then her mouth widens like a banshee and lets go a plaintive, doleful high-pitched wail. I kiss her satin cheek and whisper my love song in her ear—a version of the one I gave her at her birth when they first put her on my breast. Her single night cry is like a final resistance, a last plea against leaving the waking world for the lonely mysteries. I asked a dream therapist what she thinks babies dream and she said probably just milk, milk, milk, nurse, breast, milk. When my daughter finally succumbs to Baby Sandman— eyes deep set and heavy lidded as a newly hatched bird, elf face squished against me, breath whispery on my skin—her lips still nurse tenderly as if she is taking me and my milk with her into her silence. And I, so caught up in making sure she is not afraid, find myself no longer ruminating on my own unresolved and broken nightmares. Where I live in her dreams as comfort, food, kisses, the nest for a sweet egg—there I am safe.

Now she has taken to falling asleep in my arms, then spending half the night in her crib with the ducky bumpers and sheet, and the rest with us. Now she lies with one hand reached out to touch each of us. For half the night I have my husband's arm again and more time to finish my dreams, but I find myself listening eagerly for her soft complaining cries and the sound of her body skooching across the crib, lodging with her head in one corner where she flails her arms and legs until I reach for her. In some of the books it says to let baby settle back to sleep alone, but I never have enough discipline. I want her with me so badly that some of the old ache of birth separation returns in the middle of the night—that empty thud in the center of my body.

Guarding the Moon

One warm night she slept in just her diaper but by morning it was chilly. I brought her into our bed where we lay pressed belly to belly. Her silky milky tummy, the fragrance wafting from her pulsing fontanel, her skin as full of light as a constellation—beside such perfection I felt scarred and torn.

For years I had run for miles and miles and almost starved myself until my periods stopped. Then, after losing two babies, I prayed to be pregnant with a stomach round as the moon. Now my arms are twiggish and the skin on my belly hangs loose. Blue veins show through the skin of my breasts, and spider veins mar my legs. My hair is still shedding, my eyes tell how long I have waited for this child to come. And yet, cuddled with the most beautiful moon girl in the world, I do love my body now. Look what it has survived. Look who it has brought to us.

Dark and Light

I have always believed in the need to acknowledge life's darkness in order to fully experience love-magic. This has never been so clear to me as now, after the birth of my baby girl. And even if I attempt to deny it, the fear is always there. As I try to remember to love my body, my soul, so that I can truly love those around me, I still find myself kissing Fear's chill-bitten lips in the mirror almost every day.

I live in a city fraught with beauty, glittering with peril. I live in a cottage with an orange tree that bears giant glowing fruit, but so many fall and rot because we can't gather them all in time. The grapevines choke the wall, the pink rose struggles in the shade, the purple bursting blossom fuchsia we bought to welcome Bebe home, died after we missed watering it for one day in the frenzy of our new lives.

I feel so strange sometimes, living in this sparkler of a ravaged city, living in this body that feels too old to be raising a tiny baby, living with this man I love so much and hardly touch anymore— our hands always so full and our bodies craving sleep most of all. I heard somewhere that sleep is the sex of the new millennium. That phrase would have made me so sad at any other time of my life but now it just sounds true. I feel more passionate than ever, but I'm also too torn open to be touched. I do my yoga, but I am so much weaker now, after my body cracked like Creation to set someone free. My vision and hearing are even duller, more blurry. I feel ruined. I feel blessed. I have never had so much to write about and I have never had so little time—she cries right now; there isn't even a moment. How will I write the poems she deserves?

I want to read poetry that reflects my love and gratitude, but instead I let my fatigued brain suck up more TV than ever. After a long day of worrying alone, my eyes are strained, my mind numb, and when Busy Bee reaches behind herself to scratch and crumple every page of the book I am trying to read, I give up too easily. I watch *Buffy the Vampire Slayer* and *The X-Files* while we nurse, turning her away from the television and hitting the mute button constantly at the violent parts. I joke that if my parents read the *Odyssey* and poetry by Keats, Yeats, and Dylan Thomas to me in the womb, my daughter may recognize the voices of Mulder and Scully. She may recognize Bach but also Edith Piaf, who first made her kick in utero,

Billie Holiday, Patti Smith, Sinéad O'Connor, PJ Harvey, and Madonna.

My baby has connected me to the world of spirit, this being who was so recently all spirit, but instead of getting down on my knees at night, as I used to do, as I want to do every time I look at her, I collapse into bed, trying to send out a prayer of thanks in my mind before sleep takes me.

I look at my daughter with her luminous face, her dark blue planet eyes fringed with long tendril lashes, the goldy fuzz on top of her head that feels as airy and infinite as a cloud when I kiss it. She has two rakish bottom teeth that show when she chuckles. That laugh!

She raises her narrow shoulders, ducks her chin into its folds, closes her twinkle eyes—her whole body shakes with the force of her delight. I am stupefied with her charm. Tears of love and fear make me blind. My heart aches as if it has been torn and is trying to repair itself. My arms ache from her weight when I hold her, with longing when I don't. I have never been so happy, so relieved that she is finally here with us. I have never been so afraid.

Pain is everywhere. It hurts to grow. To get from seven pounds nine ounces, twenty-one inches to sixteen pounds four ounces, twenty-five inches in six months couldn't be an easy task. Bones lengthening, skin expanding, all those intricate organs getting bigger. The little hard knot of the umbilicus falling off; the last vestige of the con- nection to me tucked away in a plastic bag like a religious relic, leaving that vulnerable place, that sore-looking place. Even her skull slowly growing, that soft spot stretching. Tiny jagged things cutting through the soft ripe gums.

What are they? Teeth, you say? What are teeth? Never needed teeth before. What good are they in the pursuit of milk? She suckled, even in the womb. That is why she was born with a big blister in the middle of her upper lip, making it look bee stung and starletesque. Why get big? She was in me just moments ago it seems. Moving through water where nothing hurts. She still moves her hands in slow motion like a sea plant, a mermaid's tail, but now things hurt. So different from the womb where tears didn't have to fill her eyes; her world was my tears of protection and joy. The womb where food flowed at all times, where skin was always softly embraced.

Now she tries to put everything into her mouth. Sharp things, toxic things, suffocating things, choking things. My phone book pages are of special interest. Once, I looked away for a moment and discovered a huge corner missing. Imagining it blocking her throat, I felt her mouth for it and found it tucked neatly behind her upper gum. She grinned impishly at me until I pulled it out and her tears came. The same thing happened with a clothing catalog; she chomped off a piece of a male model's face, her expression placid and self-satisfied as a canary-swallowing cat, until I began to swipe the insides of her mouth. During a trip to the store she suddenly chewed off a wad of my shopping list while my back was turned. I panicked and began rummaging around in her mouth while a number of curious shoppers peered over my shoulder. When I got the paper out, one of them said cheerfully, "I thought she was chewing gum. I guess I should have said something." Gum!

I learn how you are supposed to turn a choking baby over and swat her back three times. I practice on placid, candy-pink Theodora Bear, wondering how hard to hit, wondering if I'll be able to do this. Then I hear a story about a father who had to reach his whole hand down his baby's tiny throat to retrieve the object lodged there and the swatting seems easy.

Learning to eat solid food caused a few gagging sessions that made my heart plunge. I tossed Baby Bear over my shoulder and patted her back, until she vomited a spume of milk and whatever bit of too-thick cereal I'd made. I read about wheezing, itching allergic reactions to wheat, dairy, and eggs, the toxicity for infants of something as seemingly innocuous as honey, and the choking hazard of pretty green peas. Someone even mentions that soy products can have too much natural estrogen. My milk is the only thing that feels safe, and then only if I eat a perfect, organic diet.

It seems unfair that just months after leaving the womb for a screaming, harshly lit world, babies are subjected to needles jabbed into their thighs, injections of viruses to prevent diseases like diphtheria and polio, which, thanks to these very injections, seem outdated and obsolete to most of my generation. In spite of our pediatrician's assurances, it seems I am constantly hearing terrifying stories—monkey tissue, mercury, and carcinogenic chemicals used in making the vaccines, side effects ranging from seizures to autism to SIDS. Although they deny the possibility of some of these more severe effects, the government has set up a compensation program for possible injuries sustained from the shots they advocate. How do you trust something like that? Yet I also know that as a baby I developed a sudden fever and my body began to convulse; now there is a vaccine for meningitis. I look at the scars on my ankles where I had to be fed intravenously because the veins on my arms were too tiny. I think of my mother's panic—even this many years later she can't talk about what happened without looking stricken. I finally understand why she worries so much about me when I get sick even now, how much the experience of my childhood illness changed her. How can I take any chances with my beloved's health? So we bring her to the doctor.

I hold her on my lap in her diaper while her mouth forms that curly smile for the nurse; Kewpie has no idea what is coming. Suddenly she feels pain in her tender thigh that should only know softness, kisses, warm baths, fields of flowers. I watch the bead of blood and wait, trying to breathe, to not let her feel my heart race, while the nurse applies the bandage and administers a second shot. My baby's cry is not only of pain, but of betrayal, her mouth drawn back in an incensed howl—how could you do this? We were just chatting merrily a moment ago! I take her to my breast but she can't even nurse; she keeps howling, looking up at me, needing me to know what she's been through. I whisper to her that I'm sorry, that she's all right, I know it hurts. Then she nurses passionately, gulping the milk, still sobbing. I hold her in my arms the rest of the day, looking anxiously for signs of side effects—fever or labored breathing. I wonder, have I made a mistake, is this initiation necessary? Is this a pain that could have been avoided?

Other pain is not a choice. Learning to sit up causes a few falls where she hits her head on the hard wood floor. She sees my face, distorted with worry, before I can hide it, and begins to wail. Once she fell when another child pulled a toy from her hands. I try to be calm and not swarm in waving my arms; I let our Mommy and Me yoga teacher, Rocki, help her up and give her something else to play with, gently telling the older child she must learn to share. Part of me wants to sit at my baby's side all the time, not let anyone take anything from her.

Learning to crawl is so fraught with dangers of every imaginable accident that I dread it, even as I see her frustration. She sits forlornly in yoga watching the other babies speed around the room. Sometimes she attempts to move forward and falls on her belly, arms and legs flailing, finally skooching backward instead.

Even sleep is danger. One woman I met was approached by a stranger who wanted to know if her two-month-old ever slept on her tummy— she did. The stranger said, "I'm a SIDS mom.

Make sure you don't ever let her." I am obsessed that Lambie is always flat on her back, have awakened her from a much-welcome rest if she is on her side. We wonder, somehow, if we can protect her by being close, alert, so we never really let ourselves fall too deeply into the seductive isolation of a good-night's sleep.

I try to make light of my fears with other mothers—how we are nervous wrecks, how our babies are such cute Curious Georges. We put plastic covers over the electrical outlets, bolt furniture to the floor, and put safety latches on cabinets full of deadly cleaning fluids and poisonous chemicals. We tie up the strings of venetian blinds that show a picture of a child hanging himself. Even a rubber duck is the stuff of nightmares when you imagine its plug coming out and slipping down a tiny throat. We laugh in a self-deprecating way that we are so neurotic, even about a harmless, innocent little ducky. We don't tie actual red strings on our bubela's wrists, the way those superstitious old-world Eastern Europeans once did, but we tie imaginary ones with our minds, right over the place where it looks like God already fastened a thin thread around the pudgy flesh.

One mother caught me checking my baby's breathing while she slept in her car seat. The woman looked slightly askance at my neurotic behavior, but I was sure she had done it, too. Otherwise she wouldn't have recognized the covert way I put my palm against my tiny one's soft, fragile, quiet chest to feel the reassuring rise and fall. In yoga Rocki tells us about a culture where the babies play safely at the edges of giant pits, while their parents work with knives beside them. No danger-seeking babies, no fearful worried mothers. Our nervous laughter tastes like dirty metal in our mouths.

It seems that my fear and gratitude are inextricably linked. More than ever I see how fortunate I am. The woman who comes to hold my child for two hours every couple of weeks while I write has a magic touch. Cozy Rose sleeps peacefully in the Maya wrap that this woman uses with such ease, slung on her broad body. I still haven't mastered the wrap—my child never sleeps that long with me in the day; I seem to make her loud and busy. I find myself jealous—small, shrunken, and cold. My hands are so chilly when I take my baby back that our baby-sitter laughs at me. But I learn that she cannot have a child, that she has tried for years, this woman who has such a touch, who has such warmth and soothing ways, who can will my baby to sleep for hours every time she comes. What is this gift of a child? How do I deserve it? How do I deserve my girl?

The moon knows about dark grief, danger, about the pain of growth. Ivory moon milk moon daisy moon lily moon. Ebony moon ink moon raven moon black iris ibis moon. Hidden dark-robed priestess moon. Does it hurt her to grow? Is that monthly swelling painful? How much change can one body take? And it isn't really change at all; just a change in what we perceive. The moon is always full and whole; it's just that we can't see her completely. I was startled and, at first, terrified when I learned that my hormones had caused the production of milk in my newborn daughter's nipples and given her a tiny period—not uncommon signs of the woman's body in the child's.

Does it hurt to not be seen for who you fully are, on your way to becoming?

I now measure my age by my daughter. I am thirty-seven years old, but I am also a six-month-old mother. I know I am growing from this experience, but I feel cut down. I feel like the brittle rosebushes in my neighbor's yard, violently pruned after a season of bearing heavy gorgeous baby blossoms, so that they will grow again. I don't feel like I'll grow again. I feel balding and flabby and thin. I go to my doctor for help and he says, "If you drive a car from here to New York at two hundred miles per hour, and then go to the mechanic and ask, 'Why isn't my car running?' . . . what do you expect? This body wasn't made to go at this pace." I try to explain that I can't help the pace—there never seems to be enough time to sleep or eat properly while caring for my flower. He gives me bottles of supplements and herbs, and the acupuncturist who helped me through my pregnancy covers me with healing thorn-needles. I go home and try to chew my food and breathe. I tell myself that I, too, am growing, a gibbous moon. That I, too, am like the moonflower, in a diminished cycle now, but ready to blossom full again, full of light.

One night my husband woke me with wonder in his voice. He pointed across the room to the crib. There was a mysterious radiance pouring out of it—yet the light had no visible source.

I know the baby half-moon in my house is already full. I can't see all of her yet but I believe in her, the way a part of me always believed, since I was born with my little lifetime supply of eggs, through every shattering and loss and two dilation and curettage operations to remove the fetuses whose hearts had stopped. I believed while I prayed and visualized and took my progesterone and cherry-flavored baby aspirin to help sustain the pregnancy. I always believed in my moon girl and she believes in me. When I look into her eyes I see the kind ancient wisdom of a sage who knows why she has chosen me, with all my darkness. Maybe I, dark moon, am full moon, too. I have faith in her choices; I must have faith, then, in myself.

Half

· MANNA ·

Part of what gives me continued faith in a body I doubted for so long is the milk that comes whenever it is needed. Nursing is still the sweetest thing my child and I share. Now she strokes or patty-cakes my breast and smiles slyly as she drinks. I sing to her and make her giggle and coo, never letting the flow of milk stop. I kiss the tips of her outstretched fingers and her piggy toes that she kicks up toward my mouth. Sometimes she falls asleep in my arms while nursing; when I stand she opens her mouth, latches on, and begins to suck again, eyes still closed tight.

We have nursed on a cruise ship during a wedding ceremony, wrapped in a pink pashmina shawl, and at another wedding in a hyacinth-decked arbor. On a morning glory balcony overlooking the ocean at Malibu. We have nursed in dimly lit restaurants and brightly lit dressing rooms, in shoe stores with music blaring and under shady orange trees. At book signings, art openings, and cabaret shows where she kept turning to flirt with the man behind me, flashing my breasts in the process. We often nurse while I am at my computer, becoming proficient at one-handed typing. Sometimes I've even had to run to pee, the baby kitten still attached, oblivious. No matter where we are, we make our own little world of soft peace.

Milk is the only thing that always comforts both of us; it's not just her. I used to be more tense in social situations, more self-conscious. I'd worry if I looked all right, if my husband would become intrigued with another woman. Now, with Dolly Dumpling in my arms, I am too busy with her needs to think of myself. People look at me with open, loving expressions, responding to the face tucked against my breast. I know that I will always have something to talk about, especially with the other mothers in the room—how you can't let your kids see you worry when they fall, how baby girls without hair are often mistaken for boys unless you deck them out in pink frills, how impossible it is to let your little one "cry it out," the wonder of breast-feeding. And I can always slip away to nurse, to find solace in the fastest, safest panacea, built right into my body.

When Girly-Swirl got sick with her first cold, I kept waking in the night to check her breathing. It was labored and the decongestant the doctor recommended made her vomit violently. The nurse said that breast milk squirted in her nostrils would relieve her congestion. Almost immediately upon hearing this, my milk came in more rich and constant than since she was born, engorging my breasts. When she woke in the night crying, wheezing, her miniature nostrils clogged, I took her into the bathroom and ran the hot water for steam. My husband carefully inserted the bulb syringe. She balked and cried, but when she was clear we nursed and then I put my nipple against her nostril and squirted jets of milk. She winced but didn't seem to mind that much, and it worked; she breathed well for a few hours.

What else but breast milk can clear blocked sinuses, cure eye infections, help cuts heal, comfort, ease pain, and provide perfect nutrition? Pregnancy was the first thing that made me truly see the direct link between food and sustenance. There was a time in my early twenties when I wanted to find the way to eat the least amount possible to sustain myself. Shredded wheat and nonfat milk for breakfast, a green apple for lunch, a tiny portion of tofu, rice, and vegetables for dinner. I ran around the track the moment I'd finished my meals. I got thinner and thinner. I felt a strange euphoria as I went below one hundred pounds. Down to ninety-five pounds. I had to drop out of school, leave my boyfriend, go through years of therapy. It took a long time to find a balance, but I still worried about my weight and would tend to get very thin when I needed to escape something in my life. Now here I was, pregnant, responsible for another being. I ate with extra care to vitality and health rather than calories. I consumed rich carob smoothies, tahini and banana sandwiches, avocados and omelets. I was less harsh with myself when I saw cellulite in my rear end or rolls in my abdomen.

I had a certain confidence, then, a certain brash freedom and ferocity. Once, at a restaurant, in my ninth month, I noticed a group of young-and-too-hips snickering at my protruding belly. Instead of feeling shame, I turned and lifted my shirt, jutting my tummy out in their faces. I shocked myself most of all, but it felt wonderful and they looked immediately sheepish, as if suddenly remembering that this is how most of us are actually born (though my brother suggested they might have been hatched). This belly-thrusting gesture is not something I could imagine doing now, self-conscious of even the slightly loose flesh on my abdomen that has not firmed in spite of the many sit-ups I execute most days. Still, I am reminded, when I take my hungry child in my arms to nurse, that food is, simply, to feed.

But I worry that when I wean her, I will lose this healthy connection to food. I worry that I will still like my rich foods and that when I'm no longer nursing I won't burn the calories so easily, maybe get too big. I worry that I am even having such thoughts; they fill me with shame. And this is the least of my concerns about weaning.

If I'm not breast-feeding will I still be able to in-tuit my daughter's needs in the same way? Now our stomachs ache with hunger simultaneously; my own skin feels cloying and uncomfortable when she wants to splash in a warm tub. Is there some link between the milk that flows between us and my ability to know what she needs? And what will I do to comfort her when we stop nurs-ing? Will my arms and voice and storm of kisses be enough to take away the discomfort of colds, the hurt of injections, falls, stomachaches, night-mares? Sometimes older children will come up to us and watch wistfully, hands clasped to their chests like choir boys, while we nurse. One little girl stared at my breast and repeated in a sad, soft voice, "Baby chee-chees!" Her longing to be a tiny infant, warmed and soothed by milk, made my throat dry with a melancoly thirst at the thought of having to give this up. Even breast-fed babies look at newborns wistfully as if yearning for that fearless, bundled, sleepy state. What will happen when I take the breast away? What foods will I find that heal as well as nourish?

A woman I meet tells me that she once worked at a camp for kids with cancer. One of the children there was a fifteen-year-old girl whose mother was still breast-feeding her youngest child. The mother began to nurse the older girl and her cancer went mysteriously into remission. I see in my mind that bony, long-limbed adolescent cradled awkwardly at her mother's breast. Both of them are crying. For some reason, in this vision, the girl has my face. I don't see the mother clearly, but of course she is my own,

the woman who still heals me every day. And she
is also me.

At six months my baby began to eat solids. Big
orange-pink mangoes that seem to pour juice
from their very pits. Organic little plump red-
skinned bananas with dense peachy flesh. Alli-
gator pears with their creamy green insides clinging to the smooth brown stone. Glowing papayas
full of teeny, mysterious black seeds. Cute, furred
jewel-green kiwis. Foods put on the planet just
for babies. Foods from heaven. Manna.

But not compared with what cured that fifteen-
year-old girl.

And I worry that the food Miss Mango Tango
is testing now will not be enough without my
milk, will not sustain her. She eats only a
few small bites, if any. Sometimes she hides

bits in her mouth, then starts spluttering them out with a look of glee on her face. Sometimes a spoonful of avocado makes her whole body shudder and gag. At our nine-month appointment, the nurse practitioner tells me to start introducing the foods we eat—tofu, beans, grains, vegetables—though I can't imagine that Milk Maid will like them enough to eventually give up her milky. The nurse also gives me a lecture on the importance of making mealtimes special. I agree with this and remember my childhood—gathering around the table, lighting candles, talking, reading poetry, eating the delicious risottos and enchiladas and quiches my mother made. Instead, I usually gobble down my meal of brown rice, canned beans, and steamed vegetables, then feed Baby in her high chair, or we both sprawl out on the futon with the TV on when Daddy won't be home until midnight.

I know I need to find ways to create a peaceful dining experience three times a day, though our small living room doesn't even have chairs at the second-hand drop-leaf table. Then there's the book I read about feeding your baby that warns how quickly foods can spoil—how bugs live in bags of grain, the dangers of pesticides on vegetables and mercury from fish, the rampant growth of bacteria. It's hard to imagine that nursing felt overwhelming when now it is the easiest part of feeding my sweet potato.

But my breasts are sore and drooping from her ever-increasing weight, losing their firmness, exhausted, empty. I flinch when I drive, the shoulder belt chafing my nipples. New baby teeth have pierced me, making me scream so loudly—nauseous with pain—that Milky-Silky started to cry. Now she has learned to nurse carefully, avoiding bites, but I wonder if all these sprouting teeth are a sign that I should stop nursing soon. And as she gets bigger I can't seem to eat enough to make the milk she needs. Maybe I should work harder to prepare food she likes. Even now, I'm at my computer. I tried to nurse her in my arms while I typed, but she almost hit her head on the desk so she's back in her playpen, crying. Should I be boiling organic squash or freezing applesauce in ice cube trays? Should I be feeding myself to make better milk? Sometimes, when it's time for me to prepare her food I am overcome with exhaustion. The thought of making food that she loses interest in almost immediately, that I'll probably have to discard, that might even be dangerous to her in some way, drains me weary, and then I feel guilty that I'm not being a nurturing mother.

It would almost be easier to continue our constant nursing, but what if I want another baby? Although I don't feel I have much time to wait, my doctor advises against breast-feeding while I'm pregnant. When I mention my interest in having another child to a friend, she says she wants her body back to herself for a while first. I say, "I've had my body to myself for a long, long time. Long enough." I've wanted to share it since I was in my early twenties. I've wanted babies to use it up. But now I'm almost forty, it's not so easy.

I'm going to manage, though. I'll nurse Sweet Pea and introduce as many healthy foods to her as I can. We'll pull the drop leaf out of the table, light a candle, hold hands in prayer before we eat our rice, carrots, spinach, and pink lentils. I'll get pregnant again if God intends it and if not I'll get down on my knees in gratitude for the child I do have. I'll take my calcium, eat a lot of rich things, get deeper creases around my eyes, let my breasts droop, let Baby or babies use my body up, even if there is little left of the young woman who first dreamed of being a mother. Maybe it's better to let go of her, anyway. She was haunted by so much self-hatred along with her desire for children.

I remember a boy saying to me when I was thirteen, "You'd be okay if they cut off your head." I remember hating my face. My nose. My skin. Having to go on a severe acne drug in my late twenties. On the package there was a picture of a baby with a misshapen skull; every time I took a pill I had to look at that image. The label read: "You must not take this drug while you are pregnant." I was reassured that the effects would disappear when the drug was out of my system, but I still dreaded this phantom baby. It still haunted me through my two miscarriages and even my darling's gestation. It was like an embodiment of all my self-hatred; I prayed that these feelings would not manifest themselves as a real child.

And I have been blessed with a perfect girl. I want her to know her perfection always. None of the pain of fathers who stop seeing you when you reach adolescence, of boys drawing cruel pictures, the pain that led me to drink myself into reeling blackness, get into careening cars, sleep with men who didn't love me, starve myself, imagine ways to cut myself open, trying to let out the hurt in my blood. I want to be able to transfer to my daughter, through my words, my actions, through my very milk, a message of self-love. Now, finally, I must learn to recognize my beauty so that I may protect and educate in the ways of this love, the tender beauty who came from my body into the world.

· YOGA ·

*W*atching my child learn to use her body in the world has taught me so much about my own. When she is tired she falls into a cloud of sleep as soft as she is, undisturbed by even the loudest of noises, her lips parted petals, eyes mysterious and sometimes half open, revealing a dark sapphire glimmer, like a changeling. When she is hungry she devours her milk, a ravenous celebration, making cooing noises, hums, and soft grunts all the while. She knows exactly how much she needs; when I switched calcium supplements and didn't realize I had to take more pills to get the same amount of nutrients, she increased her sucking to a practically twenty-four-hour event to get what she required until I upped my dosage. With her fluttering eyelids, tiny round nose, prominent ears, kneading fingers, demure mouth, and humming throat, she exactly resembles a lapping, purring kitten. Sometimes she pees into her diaper, grunting blissfully as she drinks. When she needs to stretch she shuts her eyes, tucks up her feet, flexes her biceps, juts out her lip, and does her Mighty Mouse impression to ease out the kinks. For her, exercise is the delight of moving her arms and legs as much as possible—kicking joyously, mischievously pulling off socks to reveal wiggly happy toes, flapping elbows like wings against her sides. When she wants air she breathes, deep from a round little belly that is softer than any silk. For her, there is no thought to the science of breath—breath, the thing I often forget when I need it most.

I have done many kinds of exercise, usually with the goal of keeping myself slender as much as healthy. I took ballet for a while as an adult, driving myself to keep up with the bone-thin, sleek, young bun-heads beside me at the barre, until I injured my knees. Sometimes I tried to remember what it felt like to dance as a child for my parents in the spotlight from my father's reading lamp. I hadn't been able to stop dancing, then. It was a bird inside of me, taking pain away, never bestowing pain.

After I had the second miscarriage I began to run. I trained with my marathoner husband, charging up steep hills until my breath seared my chest, doing intervals, entering 5Ks. Although it helped release stress, there was a ferocity to this teeth-clenching obsession. It was as if I were trying to prove something to myself. I had lost two babies, but at least I could be strong like the female athletes my husband admired. I could burn away the excess of who I was and become pure again, like a young woman with a strong heart and legs, a woman who had years of child-bearing ahead of her. I remembered running as a child, until my face was flushed, my heart leaping with pleasure as the cool wet grass tickled my feet and the smoky honeysuckle summer filled my lungs.

When I got pregnant, I began to take prenatal yoga classes. I had done some yoga in the past but never so consistently—it never distracted me enough from my life, which is the thing I often sought from a workout. But these classes—moving liquidly, stretching with the other pregnant mamas—were the most peaceful time and now, with a baby to look forward to, I needed less distraction. We breathed lavender oil and did poses with names like Dancing Goddess. Rocki ended each class with a prayer for the babies, and I imagined all of them, sleeping upside down in the big round bellies, lulled by breath, movement, and one another's presence. I felt so close to my child then. I stroked her and felt her ripple playfully, renewed by the air I was sharing with her.

While I was pregnant, exercise was not a way to sculpt my body but about nurturing the body within. After I had my yoga baby I knew that I had to nurture my own body in this same way. There was hardly time to exercise and, when I did, I needed it to serve many purposes. It had to be therapy, stress relief. It had to be a substitute for the restoration of sleep and the rejuvenation of sex.

My yogini and I began attending our Mommy and Me yoga classes when she was six weeks old. She slept in her car seat as we went up the path among the azaleas, impatiens, and the orchids in the fountain. In a small sky-lit studio sounding of wind chimes I did my practice with her beside me. Many of the women had been with us in prenatal classes. It astonished me every time I saw who had emerged from those bellies. The nodding downy heads and sleepy eyelids, the dangling stubby feet and hands, the kissy lips. When babies cried, Rocki sat on a big ball and bounced them. I looked up and saw my daughter watching me across the room, head cocked with curiosity, a gentle curve to her mouth. I wondered if I had dreamed her, if I were actually meditating, still pregnant, in a yoga class, imagining this elf with the head like the moon.

Slowly she began to move from the blanket at my side and the bouncing ball. She began to be able to sit up by herself, although she fell sometimes. She tried to crawl, inching backward instead, crying with frustration, then pushing forward, but slowly, one knee caught beneath her. Next she found she could stand propped on a block, her rear in the air. She has fallen from this position onto her back but after crying the first few times she accepts it and tumbles gracefully, the block still held at arm's length from her. When I help her walk, her feet tentatively touch the ground like delicate quilted silk fans, toes curled under, but her legs are strong, sturdy chubs. Sometimes she does a perfect Downward Dog pose. Because we go to yoga so often, it's almost as familiar to her as standing. She peeks at me, mischievous and proud, from between her legs and sometimes reaches a hand out toward me. Eventually she learns to crawl, ambling along like a pup with one foot turned in slightly as if it really wants to be standing. But she gets around this way and I can hardly remember, in just a few days, what it was like for her before she could do this. I don't think she forgets. She giggles with pleasure and freedom, in spite of the ever-present bruises mottling her chubby knees, as she finds me across the room. I share her cascade of joy but at the same time, my worry increases. When she falls against a chest of drawers in her room the bruise on her cheek is a long-lasting purple stain that I want to kiss away and that reminds me that my fears are real, sharp as wooden corners. She hardly cries.

Watching her move her body in these new ways teaches me so much. It teaches me not to be afraid to fall. It teaches me to grow in front of others, to struggle and then accept loving comfort when the struggle fails. Rocki began encouraging me to try a handstand. I have never been able to do this and even consider myself a bit phobic about it. But almost every day I practiced against a wall, feeling foolish, until now I can support myself on my little bird bone wrists and computer keyboard-gnarled fingers, while my daughter watches her funny upside-down-cake mommy. Now her papa holds her upside down and she hangs that way, grinning a crescent sparked with starry teeth. I don't know if I'll ever learn to giggle in this position, but it is inspiring. Together we are growing, outgrowing our fears.

It's hard to be afraid of looking stupid or falling on hard wood when the dangers for my princess pea are all I think about. My pain tolerance has gone way up, anyway. Maybe the racking labor helped. Maybe it is just that now I hardly feel my injuries because all I am thinking is, I'm so grateful it wasn't Pea-Wee who hit her head on that window ledge or burned her skin or cut herself.

One day when I went into the bedroom and saw her perched proudly in the crib, leaning on the railing looking over the side with a big pearly grin. We were both delighted, until I realized that the crib floor needed to be lowered—she could fall right out now. Even the thought made my insides topple.

Part of me secretly yearns for the little helpless tadpole, lying on her back waving her arms and kicking her feet, unable to go far without my help. In the same way I balk at taking her out into the world too often. But she is restless and cranky alone with me all day, with only our yoga class and walk to distract her, so I force myself to venture out. I cajole her through a smearing of sunblock that makes her look pale as a little moon-faced Kabuki babe, a little ghost girl; reload the diaper bag with changing supplies, fresh clothes, toys, and snacks; wrangle the stroller and car seat; say a prayer to the traffic gods and goddesses to surround us with light, and drive to different parks in the city. The first we visit is tiny, sawdusty, and babyless—the only people there are young film executives smoking cigarettes. But my baby has nothing to compare it to so she enjoys being out in the air, even though it's a bit smoggy, seeing the pink Chinese magnolia trees, and flirting with a nice man and his doggy.

At one park, in an upscale part of town, there are plenty of children but a snobbish attitude prevails. One mother rolls her eyes at the mention of a less chic neighborhood—"It's like a whole different world over there!"—and another looks askance when she finds I don't own a baby swing. While we are on the park swing a little boy in a cap with ear flaps comes over with his nanny, stands right in front of my girl, and starts pointing and shrieking until I take her off. The traffic is aggressive and angry on the way home and by the time I get there I am shaken and exhausted, but it was all worth it to see my daughter's smile and hear her tremulous throaty giggle each time she flew forward on the swing to meet my kiss. Another park is filled with conservative mothers and grandmothers, some of whom seem offended by my breast-feeding and possibly by my scuffed pink suede sneakers, tight jeans, and Tinker Bell "Pink Motel" glitter T-shirt. But Pinky is oblivious, breathing in the fresh dappled day, joyously leaning out of her stroller to squeal at the banks of bright pansies, and all the assorted doggies that pass us on the walkways.

Part of me wants to stay home with her, our two dogs and assorted stuffed ones, our backyard orange tree, and storybook parks. But the moon needs to grow, to dance in the sky, big white fire-fly, to hang upside down far off the ground, anchorless and free, a floating jewel belonging to everyone and no one.

· ADORNMENT ·

*A*fter my baby was born, I walked around the house with my still-distended abdomen hanging over a diaper-sized pad, no makeup, crazy hair, dripping breasts exposed, stitches holding me together. I thought, finally the self-consciousness is gone. But then the Vicoden wore off. I realized that the most beautiful part of me had left my body.

She was no longer my secret jewel, hidden in my womb, making me radiant. She had come through my cervix to grace everyone's vision, and I became suddenly invisible beside her.

My friend the Gypsy Mermaid told me, a bit pointedly, I thought, that adornment of the body exists universally in all cultures. I was irritated by what I interpreted as her implication that I should pay more attention to the superficial aspects of my appearance at this time. I became annoyed by my yoga teacher's frequent commentary on manicures and pedicures when my own cuticles lookd so ragged. I felt sapped of all energy, and it was all I could manage to eat a healthy meal or take a walk or a yoga class after I had finished nursing and changing diapers. The thought of facials, manicures, pedicures, shopping, even a haircut, made me want to shudder and weep with exhaustion.

And yet, my friends were right. Now more than ever I needed to love and honor my body.

Since the shocking breakouts I'd had as an adult I had never had cosmetic skin treatments; if I visited the dermatologist it was to have cysts punctured or get prescriptions for powerful medications. But after my daughter's birth, my skin stopped breaking out entirely. Maybe it was just my hormones settling or regular yoga or a careful avoidance of foods to which I had sensitivities.

At six weeks Beauty's skin broke out in a red pimply rash. I couldn't keep her still to file her nails short enough and she scratched herself—a jagged triangle that left a shadow on her cheek for a long time after it healed. Mortified, I immediately eliminated wheat and dairy from my diet, and the rash went away. Maybe my clearer skin was a result of that restriction. Maybe it was some symbol of a deeper self-love borne of my love for my daughter and also a sign that I had finally outgrown the adolescence that haunted me. But in any case, I finally had the opportunity to think about refinements and luxury.

The dermatologist was so infatuated with my daughter that she hardly seemed aware of me.

She said to Bambina, "How did you get such beautiful skin? I bet your mommy is going to take care of it, not let you in the sun." I am scrupulous about protecting her from UV rays but, when I was growing up, I ignored my mother's warnings and spent my summers frying with baby oil until I blistered. I was trying to burn away a layer of myself as if to find someone more lovable and lovely underneath; the freckles, lines, and wrinkles on my face and chest told that story. But with my discomfort at the dermatologist's comments came relief. Instead of being the cause of concern and attention as I had been when my skin broke out in the past, I was almost invisible, just another southern California mom with sun damage.

The same feeling of invisibility came when I took the wee kiwi with me for a haircut. I felt self-conscious about the chilling environment of most salons but my beauty consultant, Fairy Godfather Uncle Pink, suggested Goo, owned by Miss Goo, a twenty-two-year-old quick-with-the-scissors baby wrangler. In Goo, with its Pucci blue walls, I held my baby on my lap while Miss Goo cut my hair. I was ashamed of my receding postpartum hairline, hidden under layers and bangs, but no one seemed to notice or care. Goo and Uncle Pink were too enamored with the curl standing straight up on the top of Kewpie's head, the pink toes dancing to the Pink Martini CD, the chub bracelet wrists, the spray of eyelashes, and the gummy grin. After using vitamin supplements and special serums and shampoos my hair came back, but when I went for my next haircut I once again enjoyed the feeling of invisibility after so many years of self-consciousness.

The one time when I got to fully focus on myself was during the monthly manicures and pedicures

I managed to get. I understood, after the first one, why the moms in my yoga class were obsessed with this. It was about the only time I could fully inhabit my body now. Exercise was something I always shared with my baby. Making love with my husband was still a rare occurrence. I'd been jittery and self-conscious of my cuticles and calluses in the past but now, oh to sit back while two women chatted in rhythmic guttural voices, one of them stroking my hands, the other my feet. I almost fell asleep in the chair the first time. The fake cherry blossoms, the gold Buddha shrine with persimmon offerings and incense, the huge photos of hands with red lacquer talons, the glass case full of lit candy-colored bottles with names like Champagne, Bubble Gum, or U So Funny, the cheap greasy rose-scented pink lotion that was massaged into my hands and feet, all suddenly had a certain dreamy, transformational allure. I left there feeling restored, silver tipped, missing my daughter with a delicious ache, delicious because I knew I'd hold her again soon, but I'd finally had time to dream of her—the delicate scratch of her nails on my waist, the way her soft toenails peeled off to the perfect length in little crescent moons.

Once I had the pedicurist paint petals with a silver sparkle at the center on each big toe. When I showed my Flower, she squealed with delight.

One indulgence I had frequently enjoyed in the past was clothes. Even as a child, certain garments had, for me, an almost fetish magic. The purple suede lace-up shoes from London that I wore when I was ten with skirts that I convinced my mother to shorten like the minis I'd seen on Carnaby Street. The rainbow-striped sleeveless sweater covered with a smattering of rhinestones that I wore to my first rock concert. The pale peach French cotton petal-ruffled wrap skirt I wore to my sixth-grade graduation, when I still felt beautiful—at the moment before the descent into adolescence. It was a time when my hair was a pony's mane, my skin was honeysuckle flowers, I was dancing to "Turkey in the Straw" with the toughest brooding boy in my class, the skirt swirling around us. The various styles of French jeans I wore in junior high, with their intricate designs of brass buttons, laces, clips, zippers, all rather suggestive and tight; all the girls wore them with lacy T-shirts and pale suede sandals that eventually turned a lovely shade of tan, the color I wanted my skin to be. Later, clothes were a way to distinguish myself from my peers, rather than to melt in. I scoured thrift stores for silk dresses with sequin trim, old taffeta prom gowns stuffed with petticoats, a sleeveless cream wool-and-silk sweater covered with beads that I wore with black skintight ski pants and black steel-toed engineer boots. At times in my life when I was depressed, clothes lost their magic, but I knew I was doing all right, in spite of the guilt at my rampant materialism, when a pair of shoes or a new dress could make my heart beat faster or bring color to my cheeks for at least a moment. The most magical garment of all, though, was long and sleeveless with a slit up one side, a wedding gown for a mermaid, formfitting and painstakingly encrusted with pearls. I found this dress while I was waiting to hear if my first pregnancy was indeed going to miscarry—the heartbeat still wasn't detectable.

There was no heartbeat, but when I danced at my wedding the light was celestial, a miraculous clearing between two rainstorms in a canyon by the sea, and the dress I wore felt like a prayer, a collection of little eggs waiting to be fertilized, to become the pearl I was waiting for.

During my pregnancy, and after Perlita's birth, I paid little attention to clothes. I was busy preparing her cozy sleepers, her hats and booties, washing them in special allergy-free baby detergent, folding them in her drawers. But when the Gypsy Mermaid reminded me of the beauty of my own true nature, I knew I had to embellish myself again, if only to be a more generous mother.

I purchased white jeans with rhinestone trim, black Capri pants with jet beads, shirts printed with peacocks and Asian paradise gardens, a pink parasol and lotus print skirt, a skirt of bright sari silk threaded with gold, a psychedelic kimono print T-shirt. I wore high black platform sandals and pale pinkish suede boots. My baby responded to the reflection of light from the jewels on my shirts—sunbows scattering over her like fairies. She plucked with wonder at the flowers as if to try and gather a bouquet. Like a great designer she fondled the softest fabrics, held them up to examine them.

She clearly loves beauty in some innate way. Her favorite restaurant is the Vegi Tea House in Palm Desert—the low lacquer tables inlaid with abalone dragons, the red silk chairs, lotus blossoms in misty fountains, and watermelons carved with birds to resemble jade vases full of carrot and radish roses. Once she became fixated on the television screen, where a parade of chiseled male models peacocked down a runway, all cheekbones and flared nostrils, heavy eyelids, broad shoulders, slippery hips. Her heart beats faster under her thin cotton T-shirt, against my hand, when I show her Fantin-Latour's bunchy pink roses and angelic lilies; she tries to bite van Gogh's creamy swirls of white petals on a green ground; trills for Bonnard's poppies and Renoir's peaches; and reaches out, shivering, to touch eighteenth-century Dutch paintings of glossy, glassy grapes and candy-striped tulips. She points emphatically to my father's paintings—the dream-like flowers and fruits on lit-opal backgrounds, as if she recognizes them from another life.

As I saw her respond to something transcendent in color, texture, and shape, I was inspired to dress up more often. It felt like being in love for the first time. I wanted to woo her. I wanted to celebrate my love for her, show the world. I wore much less black, a staple for years, since my father's illness when I was eighteen. I wanted to wear the brightest colors, the most lush lavish flowers that told of my passion, that served as a background for the loveliest flower of all. I wanted the magic charm of fabrics and colors to transform me into a mother worthy of my daughter.

At the same time I want to convey to her that she needs nothing but herself—with only the jewels of her tears or grinning teeth, wearing just a birth-day suit—to be deserving of all love, and that adornment is just for fun. Even now we revel in dressing her in hats shaped like upside-down flower petals or strawberries, in a cozy leopard print suit with long rubber feet that dangle beyond where her actual toes fit. My beloved editor sent a pink fuzzy onesie with lavender gauze wings attached and a multicolored hand-knit cap with tassels all over it that look as if they can channel messages from the stars. My mother bought a thick white chenille dress covered with pink cabbage roses; my husband's mother sent mix-and-match pastel-striped cottons that make her granddaughter look like a jailbird elf on the lam. In the fleecy hooded jacket from her aunt she looks just like a toy lambie.

I look at the young girls singing on MTV in their sheer pants and midriff tops, their bodies undulating in striptease simulations, breasts and hair apparently enhanced. I see the parades of rear ends shaking in G-strings, anonymous young women who just want to look pretty and make a little money dancing, while little six-year-old girls all over America see them and question their own bodies, want to be models for Halloween, think they're fat, go on diets. It's hard to be a girl child. Before Twinkerbell was born, part of me wondered if it would be easier to raise a boy. But when I had the first test I wept with relief that she was healthy and with joy that she was she. Who had I yearned for ever since I was a tiny child? Who had I imagined as I dressed and walked and fed my dolls—little Leetie, Tata with the starry eyes and golden curls, and papier-mâché and glitter Picnic Rose—and poured water into Tiny Tears to make her cry? Only Plunk, named for the sound he made when he fell, was a boy. Who had haunted me as I furnished, papered, painted, and carpeted dollhouses as if preparing them for a tiny female spirit, and made up story after story about fairies and mermaids, saying them aloud as if trying to soothe some invisible babe to sleep? A little girl, my girl. I thought I'd never have her. And now here she is. I hope that her girlness will not be a pressure for her, that her self-love will dance her through.

My husband calls her the most beautiful girl in the world and her heart beats more quickly, so immediate through her thin skin, whenever she hears his voice. When she was a minute old and they took her away from me to bathe her, he stopped her tears by extending one finger for her to grasp with a grip of recognition that will bond them forever. I wonder what I would be like if my father called me beautiful from the day I was born. Would I have loved myself more? Or, when this was no longer something I could possibly believe in, would I have fallen just as hard into self-hate? Or would the sense of inner beauty have reflected out? Would I have known how to adorn and honor my body without fear throughout my life, not just sporadically and with strain? All I know is that neither my husband nor I will ever let our child be blind to her own beauty. We will encourage her joy in her reflection, that now causes her to beam, her whole body wriggling with delight. We will encourage her squeal of pleasure in her nakedness, always, the way I, as a child, was allowed to run through the house without any clothes on, giggling and loving the rush of air on my skin, before the shame of adolescence that has had a hold on me to this day.

What is perhaps most disturbing is the thought that nothing can keep pain away. My parents did love me and expressed their love generously. My father shone a spotlight on me while I danced for him; my mother always saw only my beauty, even when it was hidden in a body ravaged by adolescent sorrow. How frightening to discover that perhaps nothing we do as parents can protect.

When I was very sad about these feelings I still have, I called Nanielle, the enchantress. She had helped me with my third pregnancy, suggesting Red Clover tea, Raspberry Leaf tea, false unicorn root, sunshine, acupuncture, and an honest look at many of my fears of not being a good enough mother. She had said, with her bell-like fairy laugh, "Oh and she'll be a girl, her secret name will be Pearl!" After this prediction came true I felt I had no reason to be sad anymore, and yet I was sad, wishing to live in a body that I loved even nearly as much as the baby who had finally emerged from it. Nanielle told me to put up a picture of myself as a child, give it a name, speak to it lovingly. I found my Bubela picture. My father had taken it of me, lying down among my dolls.

My features were small and perfect, my skin was perfect—like my daughter's, not my own. All that was recognizable were my eyes, large and sad and in some way knowing. My husband looked at the picture with wonder. He called it Kitten Magic. It was as if he were seeing me again, or perhaps for the first time. I felt his love for me renewed. When my mother or a family friend tells me that I looked just like my Flower Fairy when I was a baby, or, better yet, on the rare occurrence when someone tells me that she looks like me now—somewhere around the eyes, sometimes when she smiles—I am Bubela again, my father's most beautiful girl, my husband's beloved, best of all, my daughter's mother. And what if no one tells me these things? There are plenty of times when someone will say, "How did she get so pretty?" or "Who does she look like, do you think?" or, if they don't know my husband, "She must look like her daddy?"

I remember how when she was first born, she would gaze with intense interest at her father and friends and even strangers but not at me. It worried me at first but as she molded her body to mine, reached without even looking, buried herself against me, it was as if she still believed we were one.

And now when I breathe gently on her face, she takes my breath with one deep inhale, sucks it into herself as if it gives her sustenance, as if she still gets oxygen from me as she did in the womb. She examines my body with delight, playing with strands of freshly washed hair, trying to delicately pluck a red birthmark from my leg as if it is a rare ruby. She pinches the excess flesh at my waist while she nurses, strokes my exhausted breasts with the back of her hand. No one has ever needed my body so much. Perhaps no one has ever found it so beautiful.

My doubt fades. I know I can overcome my yearning for words of praise from a father who has been gone for fifteen years. I remember that I am no longer the child who needed these words. I am Kitten Magic, Bubela, loved, loving, my daughter's mother, always.

· SONG ·

 $\mathcal{J}$ ust as girls may begin to doubt their bodies as they get older, I have heard that they may doubt their voices. My friend told me that she read about how a group of girls over a certain age will almost invariably say they can't sing when they are asked, many more than their male peers. My friend is careful not to say she can't do something in front of her three children and we discuss the need, as mothers, to get over our fears and self-consciousness. I have never sung in front of anyone since I was very little but my sweet bird doesn't mind my voice.

She uses her own voice with joyous abandon, crooning, chortling, squeaking, squealing. Sometimes she will lie for long periods of time,

waving a jingling blueberry bear, strawberry rabbit, or banana-yellow giraffe back and forth in
front of her face and singing to them in melliflu-
ous gibberish. I wonder what she is telling them.
Is she repeating the things we say to her?—"Hi,
Beautiful, I love you, you feisty girl." Is she making polite conversation—"Hey, Big Bunny, who
are you? It's fun to see you! Well, hello, little pink
sock! What are you doing here?" She blows bub-
bles, squirting spit proudly. She clucks her
tongue. She makes puckered kisses that cause us
to swoon. She will repeat one of these sounds for
a few days in a row and then switch to a new
favorite. Sometimes I am sure I detect words: hi,
yay, wow, okay, uh-oh, oh boy, but also doggy,
baby, bunny, flower, book, and ball. Slowly these
become more and more distinct. She definitely
knows Mama and Dada, which she repeats over
and over like an incantation that always brings us
to her. At first it seems that "Mama" is spoken in

times of some distress, and certainly hunger, and "Dada" only while she is playing. I'm not sure how that makes me feel—proud to be of comfort, wistful that I'm not necessarily the one in the family to be called on for fun. At about ten months Dada becomes, for a while, the word for almost everything she loves—doggy, baby, book, flower.

I can see her desire to name. She extends one finger to daintily touch the very center of the object of her affection, her eyes full of the shimmer of recognition, as she tries to find the sound for it. I think of Creation when I see babies do this. God's pointer still marks my daughter's upper lip, her pudgy elbows, and the soft plump flesh beneath each finger.

Her favorite word of all is the sound of Creation, a small "oh" full of wonder; her mouth gets tiny and round, her eyes big. Sometimes she flaps her arms and trembles with excitement. It is an expression of awe for a world full of fluffy bunnies in blue velvet bloomers; books that light up with twinkling green, gold, and red sparks from teddy bears' picnic lanterns; a green plush frog who croaks; a trilling lavender ladybug; a rocking chair covered with tea-drinking mice and elephants, with giraffes, shepherdesses, penguins, pyramids, and pagodas; camellias dripping with rain on the path to yoga; words appearing on a computer screen at the slightest touch of a hand; her own dazzling reflection popping into view; a large black box that pours out music from its mysterious innards. "Oh," in a soft, throaty whisper. Sometimes it becomes "Om"—a song of love for this world.

And the music from the boom box is the thing that generates, perhaps, the most wonder of all.

It makes her crow, waving her arms wildly in the air and kicking to the rhythms. She reaches out to the speakers, trying to grasp the ephemeral sound waves. When she was born, her favorite music was the Andean folk songs we played to calm her. I danced around with her in my arms, moving my hips. They felt so loose from labor, as if they might detach from the rest of me and samba away by themselves. She looked skyward, as if she believed music came from heaven, and stopped crying.

For me her every sound is celestial music, even her most pained cries, for they are her best way to communicate with me, still, when she needs me most. At first those cries made me shudder with her pain, made my heart race and my stomach clench with worry, but now I am so grateful for them. They can tell me more than words. They are a song, too.

During her first winter I had a series of flus. One was fever delirium and I eventually had to tell my husband, "I can't take care of her right now," words I'd never uttered before. I curled up in a shivering ball under three blankets in an eighty-degree house and realized that I had to get better fast; being sick was now almost a luxury. A month later I got a hell-pit strep throat. The throat spray I used numbed it for brief moments before it came raging back. I went on antibiotics, in spite of the problems they always caused, so that I could keep up mommy duties. Unfortunately the antibiotics made my floraless intestines more susceptible to the stomach flu that was going around. It hit suddenly. Four times, in less hours, I had to rush Teenie to her playpen, then run to the bathroom holding back the contents of my stomach, not quite making it in time. In between retches that made my whole body quake, and clammy sweat break out on my face, I called in to her, "It's all right, Sweetie, don't worry, everything is fine." She cried in a panic. When I had cleaned up as much as possible I ran in and found her on her back among equally helpless bunnies, bears, and ducks, a look of fright in her eyes that made me forget my churning, burning gut. My mother flew over on those wings of hers to hold Baby while I showered and drank sips of ginger ale. When I came back in the room after an hour or so, my child looked at me with such bouncy, toothy, gummy joy that I almost felt all better. It is still hard for me to understand how I, even with empty breasts and bruise-colored shadows under my eyes after a night of vomiting, can elicit such happiness. It is wonderful and terrifying. While I was throwing up it hit me how much she needed me, how vulnerable these moments—when I had lost control of my shuddering body—made her. But her calls from the other room reminded me that I had to get it over with, clean up, splash my face with water, smile, and go to her. Her calls will bring me back from whatever darkness for as long as it is possible.

In the same way she has brought me back from a series of nightmares: Death in a sparkling purple cloak drove an ice-cream truck full of carnival costumes into a park and took my dog Vincent away. I gave my baby sips of alcohol because someone told me to do so. I couldn't remember where I had put her down. My husband came into our hotel room and we started screaming at each other. He told me all the characteristics of his ideal woman. I pulled handfuls of hair out of my chin as we yelled. One dream was so horrific that I can never write it down. But I was roused from each one by my baby's cries for milky. She sat up, her head bent against my chest, and bleated a tiny "ow," which made me forget myself completely.

Guarding the Moon

In one dream I am balancing on a tightrope high in the glitter-strewn air, holding my newborn daughter in one hand. The instructor leans over and whispers, "That is love."

When she can't sleep in the night I sing her lullabies. I promise her the usual litany of mockingbirds and diamond rings and animals pulling carts. I sing of stars and pretty dappled ponies. There is one song my mother used to sing to me that makes me weep each time I repeat it. "I gave my love a story that had no end/I gave my love a baby with no crying/ . . . How can there be a story that has no end?/How can there be a baby with no crying?/ . . . The story of I love you, it has no end/A baby when she's sleeping, there's no crying." I remember my mother's sweet voice like golden beads and the warmth of her body as I let the song carry me to a place without tears.

Somehow, even my weak, off-key voice telling of cradles falling from treetops can soothe my lulla-baby. Although I have trusted my writer's voice since I was very young, I felt it was only worthy when it was relegated to the page, separate from a body I did not value as much. Words moved easily through my fingers but got stuck in my throat, along with the nodules that my doctor discovered on my thyroid gland when I was in my twenties. Now I am learning, as I make up lullabies about ballerinas and kangaroos, to help escort my baby to her dreams, that my body can give love through my voice as well. I, too, can sing.

· SLEEP ·

*L*ullabies send my dream girl to sleep, but not in her crib. At around six months she no longer sleeps there, but wakes with a start, shaking with tears when we set her down on her mattress rather than between us in our bed. At first we tell ourselves that it is because she has a cold—she'll be back there when she feels better. Next we blame the cold weather, but even when the heat is on she cries the second I set her on the ducky sheets. She keeps crying, wracked with sobs, her eyes shining like the glow-in-the-dark stars on the boxers I bought my (somewhat mortified) husband for Christmas. I absolutely do not have the willpower to leave her when she cries like that. I try lullabies, but she screams over my voice. I place my hand on her abdomen but she writhes and reaches her arms up for me. In a few moments I hold her and she is immediately quiet, lips in a pout, head erect, looking around with the tears still jewelling her cheeks. She sleeps peacefully in our bed, my knees curled up around her feet, her arms outstretched to touch both of us.

I am not surprised. We all need the closeness, the cuddle. Maybe my husband and I are reliving some loneliness of our babyhood cribs, when we longed to be cuddled between the two bodies we loved most, at a time when a family bed was practically taboo. We all need to reach out in the night, to feel one another's heartbeats, to hear one another's breathing and nightmare calls. My daughter and I need to nurse at a moment's notice, not to have to brave the cold, not to have to lose precious hours of sleep to find each other in the night. After all, she has only been in the world for about as long as she was a fetus in my womb. And back then our hearts wanted to beat close together, too. Instead of lying with her head down, she was in breech position for a long time. My acupuncturist said she read that this had something to do with the baby wanting to be nearer to the mother's heartbeat. Although my child assumed the correct position for her birth, there were times before that when I believed I felt her swimming upward like a mermaid toward my heart.

So our hearts still beat together, but I don't feel my husband's heartbeat anymore, or any other part of him, either.

I remember how I felt when I was pregnant—my body coursing with voluptuous blood, the most orgasmic pleasure I'd ever known. I joke with other women about our prenatal sexuality. All it takes is a knowing laugh to conjure up shared memories of what felt like insatiable desire mixed with a nagging doubt that maybe this need, these fantasies, weren't right—we were, after all, carrying our innocent precious baby, what could this ferocious sexuality be, what purpose could it serve? Perhaps it is a way to keep the father close, a celebration at the thrill of being pregnant, or just a way to release the mounting tension and fear of labor. Or maybe there is no reason at all, just pure animal urge. In any case, some of it lingered after I'd given birth. Although I was stitched together and couldn't make love, my desire for my husband, the man who had helped create this child with me after all we had been through, still shook me. But after months of illness and shattered sleep and the drain of nursing, my desire has continued to dwindle. I've spent my life craving constant touch and now, for the first time, my body winces at too much contact.

Sometimes the tension leads to raised voices, the loneliness to sullen retreats. When we do argue, our moonbeam gets very quiet or sometimes laughs nervously, a soft stuttering chuckle that stops us short, more effective than any plea. In the first weeks when we raised our voices she fell asleep suddenly, lying in my husband's palm, waking us. Although we may not touch often, she is the conduit of kisses and heartbeats. Once, when her father reached over her to massage my back, she began to pat me gently, too, with the touch of an ancient healer. When I snuggle her, she smiles in her sleep, Mona Lisa-like, as though we are dancing in her dreams.

On the fourteenth of February my husband was gone at work from seven in the morning until midnight, I was depressed, exhausted, and sick with another violent sore throat. But there was one moment when my baby just looked at me a certain way, her arms raised above her round bare tummy to yank off her strawberry cap, her eyes twinkling with blue lights, her mouth twinkling with teeth. I heard that in experiments they were able to measure love—people's brains lit up. I felt mine ignite with a thousand sparklers when I saw my perfect valentine. She is like my heart made visible; I hope such a heart beats inside of me.

I know I can wait to find my husband again. For now we have our sonnet, our love song, our wedding, our prayer, our rebirth. We witness alchemy every day. Our love for each other has taken the shape of a girl who looks like a jewel, a rose, a cloud, the moon herself.

One night I saw that celestial body low in the sky among the palm trees, perfectly full. After the rain she was mottled with wisps of cloud like a huge baroque pearl. She had drawn us out into the evening to walk, restless from the overheated house. She had called us—her daughter and her daughter's bewildered moonstruck guardian.

When my child was only a few weeks old, I woke to nurse her in the night. Desert dawns, red smog San Fernando Valley sunsets, oleanders, birthday candles, white wine in plastic cups, rhinestones fracturing light into rainbows, endless anxious freeways, glowing blue swimming pools, bleached hair, cement sizzling with a heat mirage, convertible cars, platform shoes, acne, sunburns, ice cream, jellyfish-strewn beaches, my father in a hospital like the dried and broken rose of his final still life, my mother's enveloping smile, my husband's feral eyes and gentle hands that night in his one-room apartment by the sea, when we realized, soon after we'd met, that we had both, separately, chosen the same name for the daughter we hoped someday to have. That thick bloody cord that once tied me to my baby. I saw these images in my stupor. My life flashing. I saw my death, too, in all of it.

I had felt my mortality before. When I had the biopsy on my thyroid before I discovered that the nodules were benign. When my father died. When I had to have a mammogram because of a cyst in my breast. During the ice-white searing sensations of the endometrial biopsy and the black bang of the hysteroscopy that were given to discover why I had miscarried twice. When my husband and I went for genetic counseling and I had to list all the incidents of cancer in my family. Those two D and Cs where I imagined the pain afterward was what labor would have been like.

I see the end of my life but I am not afraid now. I have finally found the one being I have always sought. Although our cord is severed I feel even closer to her. I know that among the images of burning and drowning, poisons, toxins, harsh brutal beauty and tenderness, one memory will be with me, finally—the moon having come from my womb to be placed on my breast.

Full

• BIRTHDAY •

*A*s Moon Baby's first birthday nears I see the changes come more rapidly. We are changing together, coming more fully into the light.

For me, it begins with a book. I think about how I can practically feel my brain cells dying from their TV diet. If I hadn't spent all those years by myself, pining for love and babies, reading everything, this bookless time might have been much more frustrating.

One day in a bookstore I stumble upon an edition of collected poems. On the cover a woman stretches out her long legs and sandaled feet and gazes with light sad eyes. Inside, she writes of hospital rooms, daughters, clowns, witches, dolls, trees, tumors, eyeballs, guns, crosses. I never read much of her in college. The gods were big marble heads without bodies, men with husk hearts, broken statues, crisp shards of fractured words. I read now these confessions of the body, informed by what I have just been through—this birth—and even the most pained poems uplift me. Because I am reading, because I have images and sounds in me again. I think that poetry is perfect for women raising children, with just bits of time and such need to connect to other women out of the isolation of motherhood. I watch my daughter nibbling on *The Runaway Bunny* and *Pat the Pony*, trying to devour them, and I understand—this is food.

Her diet has changed, too. She still nurses ravenously a few times a day, pumping her legs, thumping my chest, blithely tickling my armpit as she inhales the milk. At night she wakes at least twice for more, but sometimes it is just for comfort, a quick reminder that I am still here for her. We probably won't wean from each other for a long time, but at least she is relishing other food experiences as well, and I am encouraged to cook.

Although she meticulously picks up rice cake crumbs from among the wreckage of her discarded meal, savoring each one as if it is the most nourishing sublime morsel, there are days when she also smacks her lips for baked salmon, steamed broccoli, hard-boiled egg, and tofu chunks, and she slurps up pasta and seaweed strands. The sight of the bursting sunny oranges that grow on our tree make her pucker up as if for a kiss and flap her arms with excitement, calling, "Ah ah." She sucks juice noisily, lustily from her sippy cup, otherwise known as pitta-pitta-pitta. When she devours my black bean or broccoli soup, my hummus, molasses banana bread, or apple-juice-sweetened carrot cake, I consider it one of my life's greatest achievements.

We go to our favorite sushi restaurant, Noshi, where she lounges in the high chair, leaning on her elbow like a gangster or movie mogul, pleasure-drunk on fistfuls of squeaky-clean white rose rice that sticks to her clothes, bright green edamame, and slippery bits of avocado. At another Japanese place, the waitresses giggle about the soba noodles hanging from Baby Bird's mouth, like worms in a beak. Later, we find dried noodles everywhere—caught in her diapers, curled in the bedsheets. I remember how she first leaped in the womb when I listened to Edith Piaf after a soba dinner. Noodle Girl. We have a birthday dinner for my husband at an Italian restaurant and she daintily picks up and chews on penne, pinkie finger extended, and charms both her handsome uncles to distraction.

The next morning I wake to nurse my social butterfly and when she falls back to sleep, I get up to put in my diaphragm and slip onto my husband's side of the bed. I don't know if it is the red wine and salmon dinner, the poetry I'd been reading, the lack of TV, or the fact that Bubela slept better, but my husband and I make love and it doesn't even hurt, though the next day my hips feel strange, displaced and pleasantly sore. When I get my period two days later—that almost forgotten backache, that iron-scented staining that never made so much sense before—I think about having a second child after all.

There's that soft phantom space in our lives still, though it doesn't throb like the space that my daughter has now filled. When I was pregnant the first time I felt it was a boy. My husband and I had already chosen to name him after both of our mothers' beloved tender fathers. I was imbued with this boy's spirit; I felt his gestures in my own hands, his sweet nature churning my stomach and singing my heart like a birthday. I wrote him love poems every night. I loved him, and not just because he was my baby, but for his singular soul, just as I loved my daughter in the womb, though, having known loss and fearing more of it, I did not write to her. I remember the night when I woke, after bleeding slow drops for a week, and heard a voice whispering good-bye. It sounded like the spirit of the eucalyptus trees— thin, silver-green in moonlight. I felt the child leaving us. Part of me yearns to find him again. Part of me yearns for a second daughter, named for a polished green gemstone this time, not a fragrant white flower. I imagine myself with my two girls, dancing in a circle, brushing one another's hair, sleeping like a pile of kittens, all of us freed somehow, from our loneliness, by the magic number three, number of pyramids and tea parties.

I wonder how my firstborn will feel about a sibling, boy or girl. I know that she is tender with other children. In yoga she caresses two-year-old Devon's shiny blond hair and baby-doll face, reads books with one-year-old Kayla, and sits quietly chewing Elmo beside six-month-old Baby Shira. Yoga-Baby Emerson often steals my girl's frilly socks and runs around with one in each hand, waving them like flags and crowing. On the day this sturdy, seemingly invincible one-year-old bumped himself hard enough to cry, she crawled over to his mama and put a worried hand on her leg, cocking her own head like a sad pup, leaning over to try to see if he was all right. Tinier Yoga-Baby Emerson, with the dreamy nursery-rhyme eyes and smile, lies on his belly wiggling with frustration, ready to crawl. My yoga babe goes over to him and tries to pat his big flower head, as if to tell him she understands, she's been there, you'll be cruising with me soon, bud.

I know a sibling can be a challenge, though, even for the most loving little Mamala who tenderly kisses and licks her dolly and tries to console her friends. What if she is still sleeping in our bed when a new child comes along to usurp the cozy place between our bodies? What if she's still nursing? Can you nurse two babies at once? Maybe some earth mother with abundant breasts, but can I? Is another child even possible from this body?

My doubts are reinforced when we go for our one-year checkup. Everything seems perfect. Everyone in the office coos over the Kewpie curl, the smile now made up of ten tiny pearly whites, the way the sweet pea stands up to try to kiss her reflection in the mirror. Then our nurse practitioner notices that Miss Kiss's hair seems very dry at the back of her head. She suggests I add more fat to her diet, though I've been trying to use lots of avocado and flaxseed oil, and then orders a blood test. Another nurse pricks those tiny toes, then comes back in and announces, "Don't leave yet!" with alarm in her voice. I feel my blood drain with worry. Baby is extremely anemic. The nurse says this condition can lead to slow brain development and susceptibility to illness—I think of our series of colds all winter. She wants us to administer iron drops, but also to add calf's liver and liverwurst to Bambina's diet.

I feel that strange inadequacy again. I was anemic for a while during the pregnancy. Maybe my milk isn't good enough, not to mention my cooking and cajoling skills at the dinner table. How will I prepare a food that used to make me weep when I saw it glistening red-brown slime in the butcher shop or even when I smelled it cooking on Jewish holidays? How will I make something for my child if I can't convince myself that it is really healthy? I decide to use the drops and try to find semi-vegetarian alternatives, but the worry lodges itself in my throat. The next morning I prepare scrambled eggs, steamed broccoli, molasses bread, iron-fortified cereal, and orange juice sprinkled with green powder from my vegetable supplement capsules. My picky eater eats one bit of a broccoli floweret, some crumbs of bread, a spoonful of cereal, and drinks her juice, all the while squeaking and pointing insistently at the package of zero percent iron rice cakes that I forgot to hide. I coat a few with molasses but she only likes them plain and I know it's time for the drops, that, I'm dismayed to find, contain alcohol, sugar, and preservatives. It is challenging to even get the exact amount in the dropper. Worrying about iron toxicity and poking my baby, I take a deep breath and push the drops into her mouth when she opens it to cry in protest. We end up back in the safety of our pink rocking chair, nursing, comforting each other.

A few weeks later her hair still seems dry, her appetite hasn't improved much, and sometimes she looks very pale, with shadows under her eyes. My mother comes over with calf's liver from the health-food store, sauteed with onions and served with chopped egg and jasmine rice, and her granddaughter eats it with pleasure. My mom has given me countless things in my life, but this may be one of the biggest gifts of all. The twisting in my stomach releases as I watch Baby eat with both hands, eyes glazed. Unfortunately, when I face my phobias and try to cook a small piece of organic liver, I'm so worried about serving it too rare that I end up charring it inedible.

I worry about my ability to feed even one child, and I feel less sure about getting pregnant again. I have flashbacks of trying to conceive after the miscarriages—one fertility expert wanted me to inject my abdomen with a needle twice a day for the entire pregnancy. Though I chose not to do this, I still wince, not only for myself, but when I think of the baby trying to grow there. Now my doctor recommends that I continue to wait to conceive while I'm this worn out, especially if I'm going to keep nursing. I look for ways to restore myself.

Our baby-sitter became unavailable when Sugar Plumpkin was about nine months old, so we've been trying to manage on our own since. One subsequent sitter looked around our home, askance, said she felt sorry for our child (having to learn to crawl on less-than-immaculate hardwood floors among two dogs, I presume), and insisted that she couldn't watch her in this environment. I still need my girl at home with me as much as possible, while I write, so I decide against taking her to the sitter's house. I try out another lady who keeps saying forlornly that we live so far away but she really needs the money; then she gets lost twice and ends up going home. A third sitter never bothers to come or call on the day we expect her.

There are times when Vincent has diarrhea or vomits on the floor. Once Thumper took off over the backyard fence and was found trembling in the middle of a crowded intersection. The second time she ran away she came back in half an hour, arriving inexplicably on our doorstep with a cooked, sliced ham, three times the size of her head, hanging proudly from her mouth.

Our baby gets more bruises on her head from falling on the floor, sobs hysterically if she's not being held. She gets another cold, gets a fever so high that I think I have one when I sleep beside her incandescent body. I have to get over yet another phobia and take her temperature. My

pediatrician insists that the underarm thermome-
ters aren't reliable. I'm not sure if I actually
remember the discomfort and humiliation of having a thermometer in my bottom, or if I'm just
identifying, but I've never been able to do this
before. Now I force myself. And I panic, watching the digital numbers soar, until I realize I'm
supposed to subtract .9 degrees.

By late afternoon on most days my skin is itching
and I'm insatiably hungry after nursing for hours at
a time. I yearn for a bath to soothe my sore breasts,
a meal chewed rather than gulped, or at least a few
minutes to pee without my child screaming from
her playpen in the next room or following me into
the bathroom to stand balancing against the tub,
her head precariously close to the tile.

My mother comes when she can, all smiles and
soups and soft cotton clothes and dolls and bears,

nontoxic chew toys and baby safety devices, in addition to the liver that I now appreciate for its iron content, rather than abhor. I want to collapse with relief and sleep for hours but there's too much to do. I hire a housekeeper who finds time in her six-day work week to do some kind of crazy magic, making everything gleam in five hours, changing the very air of our little crowded house. A clean floor never seemed so important, so spiritually soothing, even, when I know I can put Miss Creepy Crawler down on it without worries, though it's Two-Dog-dirty again in moments.

My husband is always trying to get me to nap when he is home, but I never feel I can afford to use the time that way. He says that getting me or our daughter to rest is worse than trying to catch a tiger by the tail. I think that her reason for not napping has to do with the need to see everything; as she starts to close her eyes she opens them suddenly and looks around to make sure she hasn't missed the fun. When I try to nap, I jump up to chase dust balls instead, worrying that I should be writing this book.

Finally I do go for a manicure, pedicure, and wax to help myself recover from a night of little sleep, but afterward I feel worse. While waxing my "bikini area" the beautician scrutinizes my face and says, "Oh, you waited a long time to have a baby. Why? You married late?" So much for the enchantment of corner beauty parlors with their shrines and pretty paints. I try not to start crying as she rips out hair from the most vulnerable part of my body.

I've been called oversensitive and lately, though I don't have time to get upset as often, it seems to cut deeper. When the interviewer asks me if I'm ever going to write a real book, I get off the phone and burst into tears in my husband's arms. I don't know if I imagined the interviewer's anti-Semitism or not, but I didn't imagine the chilling hostility.

One of my friends told me that her father's parents were Holocaust survivors who lost three children before giving birth to him. It still shocks me how recently this thing happened, and every time anyone mentions it I want to pull my child to my breast and cover her eyes and ears. See no evil, hear no evil, know not the evils of this world, never leave this safe place we have made for you. Flowers and doggies and bunnies and bears and balls. Giving birth, being a mama, spending time with other mothers who have young children, writing about my daughter—all these things have opened me up, dissolved my defenses. Sometimes I feel like one of the oranges from the tree—falling off so easily into outstretched hands—peeled and sectioned, the insides translucent and wet, waiting to be consumed. I forget the harshness of the world.

My husband has some time off work, so we go to Palm Desert where his parents have a condo. We came, almost a year ago, to this hot, pink-sand valley among the cool blue snow mountains to heal from the series of tests we'd taken to determine why we couldn't hold a pregnancy. The palm trees and pools were shivery metallic, glittering with wind and sun. On the way to the Jacuzzi we saw something moving on my husband's bare shoulder. It was a pair of white butterflies mating in a delicate frenzy. We took it as a sign, a kind of annunciation, even, and conceived our daughter a few days later, back in Los Angeles.

That was a trip for three—us and our little boy, Vincent. We've been back a few times since and now we go to see Grammy and Grampa with Two Dogs and the baby who was so recently only a flutter of white wings in our hearts. In the desert she chatters all the time, pointing at everything and asking, "What dat? What dat?" Window, door, light, flowers, picture. Everything seems to shine with newness, rediscovered like a word in a perfect poem. She crawls around faster than ever and practices dainty tippy-toe steps while holding my hands in the carpeted rooms. The mirrored wall is of special interest, maybe because we don't have a full-length mirror at home. I actually prefer avoiding my reflection and the wasted moments of self-scrutiny but, for her, a mirror is a looking glass, a plaything, a wonder, an alternate universe, a friend. She tries to lick the baby girl with raspberry-stained lips. When she bumps her head she bravely continues to explore, until her hands and feet are dusty, and we bathe her wriggly busy tadpole body in

the kitchen sink, though she barely fits there anymore. After, we go to the ornate Vegi Tea House,
for their miniature boats full of farm-grown vegetables, so fresh they almost buzz, intoxicating
soy crepes, fresh-squeezed watermelon juice, and
brown rice in balsa wood boxes. Our desert rose
zestfully eats bits of bean sprouts, zucchini, carrots, and mushrooms. At home I nurse her to
sleep and the curls at the back of her neck get
damp with our sweat; her baby flower fragrance
floats up. I put her down next to me and she lies
with her arms flung out as if to embrace the
whole hyacinth-scented, watermelon-colored
world.

We all sleep better here, even Two Dogs are less
restless. My husband and I are calmer, too,
and even have some moments alone together. We
run around the golf course—that strange phe-
nomenon of green slopes, petunias, pansies,

snapdragons, hibiscus, oleander, and bougainvillea in the midst of such an arid world. I didn't think I had any strength to run but I manage it, encouraged by his voice and stride, by the burnished air and glimpses of Baby in her carriage as Grammy walks her. Afterward, we slide our aching bodies into the rumbling spa water, that little pool under the purple-flowering jacaranda and chocolate-scented carob trees, where we once kissed, dreaming of a baby moon. We can hold each other up in the water, hold each other as we do our child, bundled and weightless like newborns. Some of that feeling comes home in our bones. On the drive back Vincent licks Little's bare berry toes and she giggles extravagantly in between guzzles on her sippy cup and little clucking songs. They fall asleep, his chin on her bare cherub leg, her brow smooth with dreams of lit windows, flowery water.

I feel better after the desert but in a week I'm sick again. Fortunately my child only gets a cold; I wonder if all my illnesses are a way to help her build her immunities. One night, when each minute of sleep is like a bite of food to a starving belly, I feel her turn onto her side, put her arms around my neck, and hoist herself up onto my breast. It is as if I am being emptied of all the life force left in my body. Every nerve ending burns. I want to sleep so badly. And yet here she is finding me, hugging me, kitten-soft, daffodil-sweet, fighting illness with the milk from my feverish body as her weapon.

I think of my own mother. She didn't sleep for two days and nights during my labor and stayed over for a week after Lambie's birth. Once I woke and found her sleeping sitting up with her feet on the floor, one arm cradled in the other. She had fallen earlier that day and couldn't lie flat, but she hadn't wanted to worry us. My mother has done things like this for me every day of my life. Sometimes I used to think she was an angel—truly. This light comes out of her, just like it comes out of her granddaughter, a pearly luminescence. People note the similarities in their broad, smiling, radiant faces and light-filled eyes. I still think my mother is an angel but now, also, I understand how the love a mama feels can make her give up food and sleep and peace and parts of her body. And much of what might have seemed like a sacrifice before actually only enriches my life.

When my husband and I would rather stay home and rest, we drive up the coast, lather our girl with sunblock, and let her gambol on sand dunes among purple wildflowers, touch her curious curling toes into an ocean that has never seemed so vast to me. In spite of exhausting worries about sunburn and insect bites and germs and accidents, I find myself rejuvenated afterward.

I take the 'bina on hour-long walks, down busy boulevards, over curbs without ramps, past freeway entrances, to get to the neighborhood of Tudor homes and gardenia gardens across the park bridge, remembering how I used to hold my breath on a stroll down the block. The harshly pruned roses in my neighbor's yard are huge now—peach, pink, orange, red, wearing necklaces of purple pansies. "Wowa! Wowa!" my girl cries when we pass, as if greeting old friends. Patting the stroller bar, leaning forward to catch everything. "Ma-ma Ma-ma-ma," she sings as she rolls along, as if thanking me for these adventures.

I remember times in my life when I was too self-conscious to sing "Happy Birthday," but now we buy a tiny tambourine and go to music classes, at a friend's sunny glass hideaway apartment tucked into a hillside, and I join in with the other mothers, in spite of my canker sore, which flames when my tooth scrapes it, and my embarrassingly off-key voice. My child smiling in a sunny singing circle makes me forget myself again. I take her swimming at a friend's pool, too delighted with her mer-baby frolics to think about how my pale body looks in a bathing suit. After a week of brutal fourteen-hour days my husband manages to spend his weekend picking us up from yoga, taking us out for spinach omelets and pumpkin muffins, and walking in the park on the cliffs above the sea.

Having a baby makes me taste food I once just swallowed, or sometimes choked down, smell the fresh salt, cut grass, barbecue smoke, and roses in the air; it makes me see the parade of funny dogs, the towering palm trees, green lawns, the silver-blue sheen of water. Bunnies really hop and their noses twitch, twitch, twitch. Nine baby ducks swim with their mama in a pond—damp, mottled-brown extensions of her own body. Although my duckling often claps her hands and squeals, sometimes it seems as if she is showing me a world she already knows profoundly well. At our veterinarian's ranch, I showed my daughter the horses in their stalls. I felt the heady rush of their huge silent mass, the grace of acceptance in their stance. As she stared at them without blinking and they stared back, eyes welling with wisdom, quiet ferocity, and a strange recognition, I felt that it was perhaps she who was showing me.

And she has shown me my best self. It is as if she chose me in spite of everything, in spite of my jealousies and eating disorders and skin reactions and my multiply fractured heart. Somehow, in spite of all that, she saw someone to carry her here.

And she has shown me to others.

In every childhood photo of my brother and me, I am gazing up at him with adoration, while part of him always seems to look away. Now he buys my daughter seven bunnies in hats to go with the seven sweater bears—he says he can't go into a store without picking up a fluffy guy for her. He turns down an acting job on a soap opera in New York, in part, he says, so he won't have to leave her. When she was born he squinted at her, frowned, and asked if I thought she resembled me at all. Now he says, "She has those veins showing through the skin like we do." He says to me dreamily, remembering, "She reminds me of you when you were a baby."

When the beautiful girl left my body, I had to share her with her father so suddenly, and share him, of course, with her. Sometimes I woke at night, head bursting with pain, an aftereffect of the drugs I'd been given during labor. At these times, while my husband slept, when my daughter turned away in the bed, Fear fingered me and I felt that I was becoming invisible. Sometimes, now, I am too exhausted to even greet my husband with the smiles and hugs he deserves; his daughter trills her "hi" and practically shivers with delight when he enters the room.

I know he understands my sullen states, as I understand his occasional flares of anger. In our kiss is unspoken forgiveness for behavior borne of frustration and fatigue. When Baby cries for me and can only be consoled at my breast, my husband says, "She's infused with Kitten Magic. Always remember rule number one: never doubt the magic." He says to her: "You love your mom. You love your mom, don't you?" No other expression could tell so much of his own feelings for me, his most beautiful girl's mama, his beloved child's beloved. "What a pair," he says, seeing us both.

One evening, on Passover, my mother and I take a walk with the baby and talk about what would free us, how to clear out our cluttered lives. My mama says there are certain things she can't give up—art books of my dad's, letters from her father—but she wants me to feel free to dispose of them when she "flies away." She says, "I've never talked about this before but I would like to be cremated." I don't want her to say these words, but somehow it helps. The unspoken is much worse in a way. I remember when my mother told me my grandmother had died. I was very young but I still recall, perfectly, the overcast afternoon, smelling of moist bitter trees, and how we both cried, our tears mingling, drenching my mother's braid and her camel corduroy coat with the toggle buttons. I wasn't that close to my grandmother, not the way my child already is to hers, but I understood what was happening enough to know that someday I would lose my mother, too. Perhaps after having my child I am now better able to accept my mortality and even my mother's, knowing that our feelings for each other live on in this girl, this Tweety Bird, Giggle Bean, Hug Bug, this Love of Our Lives.

But as much as I have found peace, pain continues, as it does. This book isn't a novel, after all; there's no resolution for life. But I'll keep trying. If this was a novel the mama would no longer use self-hatred as a way to ward off fears of losing her loved ones, as a way to ward off death. She would see her beauty, strange and changeable, see that she is an elf boy and a fairy with the eyes of a crone and the eyes of a maiden, a nuzzling nose, a mouth full of kisses, nourishing breasts, legs that can still run. She would honor her skin, that she once despised for its pallor, realizing that it was once moon-girl beautiful and now lit with love, scarred with compassion. It would seem, by the fact that all novels end, that she will see herself this way forever.

Instead I see my daughter.

She lies in the crook of my arm, curled into my body as if she is still living there, though our cord is long gone from her silky milk-full pink-pearl belly. Her eyelids are just like two Picasso doves, flying above her wide mouth and tiny pointed chin. She has that show-stopping

Kewpie curl on the top of her head and new tender tendrils forming at the base of her neck. Her skin pulses with light like the heartbeat pulse I feel at her throat.

Charm School wakes suddenly, opens her eyes wide, makes her mouth into that little *o* and points at something in the room: "What dat? Aka-ta," she cries—"Look at that!" Or she turns to her daddy's side of the bed when he's already up and asks, "Where Dada?" When I lift her in my arms to nurse she immediately stops complaining and says, "Op," a celebration of being upright as much as a statement. She hoists to standing ("Op op op") and holds herself steady for a few seconds, grinning, swaying her hips, waving her hands in the air, and proudly imitating our praises ("ga ga ga" for "good") before plopping to her bottom or gently lowering herself back down into a squat. She crawls rhythmically, fast, hands patting the floor, crying, "Go go go go go," like a chant of determination. She waves, fingers like petals in a breeze, cocking her head all the way to her shoulder and grinning shyly, delighted, and perhaps relieved, to be able to communicate this way at last. Her "hi" is a sigh, melty as chocolate. She points to flowers in gardens and prints of blossoms on shawls, on walls, on bedspreads. "Wowa! Wowa!" "Bir," she croons to the sparrows on the path, "bir, bir bir." "Ba!" she squeals, running after the pastel plush Pooh Bear ball with the bell inside, or pointing to a row of round white paper lanterns. When she bumps her head, she rubs it and murmurs a heartaching "ow." When I ask her where her mouth is, she tentatively inserts three fingers as if to test out her theory. When I ask where her hair is, she reaches behind to the back of her head and pats softly as if petting a baby animal.

She takes her pursed-lipped baby doll in her arms and passionately covers its mouth with her own when I say, "Kiss kiss." "Bay!" she exclaims. "Dada" is a song of pure delight, but sometimes she sings it wistfully, pointing at every man in the restaurant while the real thing is off at work. When she calls "Mama," I want to squeak the way she does when she greets her baby. One night, as she lay beside me after nursing, she said my name softly, hoarsely, peacefully in her sleep, not needing anything, just dreaming.

I see her in all her morning-glory and night-blooming splendor, healing those who need it most. The abrasive soften in her presence, the depressed light up. Once a smiling boy emerged from the concave face of an elderly gentleman in a wheelchair who passed her on our walk by the sea. Countless times, people I would never exchange a word with otherwise, fall into rhapsodies about her.

During her birthday fiesta, her day for gifts, she gives to everyone. She wears the chenille cabbage rose dress from Grandma that serves as a perfect mop when she crawls in zigzags across the floor. Crawling to her daddy, she stands before him, waving a photo of a newborn clinging to a man's finger, just the way she grasped her father's finger one year ago this day. It is the clearest communication of her love she could possibly give to him and, overcome, he has to hand the video camera to me. She kisses my shyest friend, cuddles for equal amounts of time with both grandmas, bounces in my arms when she sees the heart-shaped, fruit-juice sweetened, tiny-rose-decorated cake I overcame my baking phobia to make for her.

We all glow with her reflection. Uncle Pink gave me a pink rose and an elixir in a Japanese garden after my miscarriage and dreamed of Baby Buddha before she was born, when my dreams were only of disease and darkness. When I speak of the effect she has on people he asks me, "You aren't surprised?" Of course not—think of how she came to me, my flower of flowers, my ice-cream bells, my heart's fairy, Kwan Yin Goddess, rising out of the wreckage of loss with her smooth moon head and her azure forever gaze. She was born in the Chinese year of the Golden Dragon and such babies are said to bring good fortune to their families. When a project I've been working on for twelve years finally comes to fruition days before my dragon's birthday, Nanielle says, "I'm going to tell you something in code—Pearl did this." Of course. Ladybugs decked me like jewels while I carried her inside, butterflies made love on her father's bare sunny shoulders, two dogs found their soul mates in our home, red-and-white striped amaryllis and purple-pink evening primrose bloomed overnight on the day she was born, birds sing her lullabies at midnight, bunnies and bears and bouquets and books parade to our door. When she was just months old and I answered her sneeze with "God bless you," she smiled that dreamy beam as if she understood the phrase perfectly.

One night she pointed to the moon, full-blown like a white poppy floating above the palms in the blue-tinged evening sky. "What dat? What dat? Ah?" *Ah*—her word for lights and eggs and oranges. "It's the moon, darling one." She cried when I tried to bring her back inside. Pointing to the porch light, "Ah. Ah." And then, reaching up to touch the biggest night-light of all. "Mmm Mama," my child said. "Mama."

Though pain and self-doubt continue, the salt-packed feeling of tears in my throat is dissolving. My daughter, my Jasmine Angelina, has blessed me, has healed my greatest wound—my lifelong need for her—with, simply, her arrival.

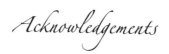

Acknowledgements

Thanks to Lydia Wills, a true moon guardian, for encouraging me to write this in the first place, Joanna Cotler for guiding me with such wisdom and love, and Megan Newman for making it happen. I'd also like to thank my friends Tracey and Sarah Porter, Paul Monroe, Molly Bendall, Debbie McAfee, Hillary Carlip, and the Masterminders—Andrea Beard, Bonnie and Shira Goldstein, Lisa and Kayla Klein-Wolf, Carmen Staton and Hannah Scott, Simone and Jana Heckerman, Stella Michaelis and Lara Foley, Michele and Jacqueline Weeger, Rocki Graham, and all the Yoga Baby moms and kids for tremendous support, information, and a treasured community. My thanks to Angela Cheng Caplan, Paula Shuster, Jessica Shulsinger, Sita White, Jodi Peikoff, and Alicia Mikles for making my work a joy. Dr. Soram Singh Khalsa, Dr. Hal Danzer, Dr. Paula Goldstein, Dr. Stephen Rabin, Dr. Paul Crane, Behnaz Forat, Nanielle Devreaux, Lew Fein, Julie Freitas, Dr. Linda Nussbaum, Dr. Jay Gordon, Michael and Morningstar— thank you for your healing. Finally, I want to express my loving gratitude to Alice and Bob Schuette, Robin Schuette, Jay Schuette, Gregg Marx, and especially Gilda Block, Chris Schuette, Samuel Alexander Schuette, and Jasmine Angelina Schuette, who makes everything and anything possible.